Renal Diet and Cookbook:

Delicious and Healthy Recipes for Managing Kidney Disease

Dr. Louvenia W. Williamson

TABLE OF CONTENTS.

CHAPTER ONE

1.0 Introduction

1.1 What is a Renal Diet?

1.2 Advantages of Following a Renal Diet

1.3 How to Use This Cookbook

CHAPTER TWO

2.0 Renal Diet Basics

2.1 Understanding Kidney Disease

2.2 Nutritional Needs for Renal Diets

2.3 Foods to Limit or Avoid

2.4 Items to Incorporate into a Renal Diet

CHAPTER THREE
3.0 Morning Recipes

3.1 oatmeal

3.1.1 Apple oatmeal custard:

3.1.2 Strawberry and peanut oatmeal bowl

3.1.3 Blueberry overnight oats

3.1.4 Strawberry chia overnight Oats

3.1.5 Strawberry chia overnight oats

3.1.6 Oatmeal porridge

3.2 Scrambled Eggs

3.2.1 Stuffed vegetable eggs

3.2.2 Scrambled eggs with kidney beans
and cheddar

3.2.3 Festive eggs scramble

3.2.4 Tofu breakfast scramble

3.2.5 Scrambled eggs, smashed avocado, and bean breakfast

3.3 smoothies

3.3.1 Blueberry blast smoothie

3.3.2 Pineapple protein smoothie

3.3.3 Fruity smoothie

3.3.4 Blended berry smoothie

3.3.5 Peach High-Protein Smoothie

3.3.6 Strawberry High-Protein Smoothie

3.4 Toast

3.4.1 Sprouted-grain toast with peanut butter and banana

3.4.2 Whole grain peanut butter and fruit toast

3.4.3 Peanut butter and banana on toast

3.4.4 Peanut butter fruit toast

3.5 Bagel with Cream Cheese

3.5.1 Bagel with creamy cheese

3.5.2 Bagel with avocado and creamy cheese

CHAPTER FOUR

4.0 Snack Recipes

4.1 Cranberry dip with fresh fruits

4.2 Tender ginger biscuits

4.3 Delicious popcorn balls

4.4 Cucumber with sour cream

4.5 Hungarian sour cherry soup

4.6 Sweet and sour meatballs

4.7 Hot cornbread

4.8 Hot crunchy and munch snack combo

4.9 Sweet and spicy tortilla chips

4.10 Addictive pretzels

4.11 Shrimp spray with crackers

4.12 Wonton quiche minis

CHAPTER FIVE

5.0 Salad and Appetizer Recipes

5.1 Cool coconut marshmallow salad

5.2 Pineapple coleslaw

5.3 Pineapple coleslaw

5.4 Low-salt macaroni and cheese

5.5 Low-salt macaroni and cheese

5.6 Buffalo chicken salad cucumber cups

5.7 Chili cornbread casserole

5.8 Caribbean lime shrimp salad

5.9 Creamy caesar salad-keto renal

5.10 Blackberry spinach salad

CHAPTER SIX

<u>6.0 Main Dish Recipes</u>

<u>6.1 Grain hot cereal</u>

<u>6.2 Baba ghanoush</u>

<u>6.3 Beef and vegetable kebabs</u>

<u>6.4 Broccoli, garlic, and rigatoni</u>

<u>6.5 Chicken brats</u>

<u>6.6 Chicken salad with pineapple balsamic vinaigrette</u>

<u>6.7 Corn tamales with avocado-tomatillo salsa</u>

<u>6.8 Fettuccine with clams, brazil, tomato, corn, and garlic</u>

<u>6.9 Fish tacos with tomatillo sauce</u>
<u>6.10 Grilled pork fajitas</u>

6.11 Mango salsa pizza

6.12 Spaghetti with spinach, garbanzos, and raisins

6.13 Rice noodles with spring veggies

6.14 Smoky bean and mushroom cornucopia

6.15 Spinach and mushrooms frittata

6.16 Vegetable stir-fry

CHAPTER SEVEN

7.0 Side Dish Recipes

7.1 Mushroom and garlic spaghetti meal

7.2 fried rice

7.3 Mushroom asparagus pasta

7.4 Hot chicken penne

7.5 beautiful lemon rice with veggies

7.6 Oven-baked green bean fries

7.7 chicken and wild rice casserole with butternut squash

CHAPTER EIGHT

8.0 Dessert Recipes

8.1 Berries homemade popsicles

8.2 Pumpkin strudel

8.3 Delicious cherry cobbler

8.4 Little pineapple upside-down cake

CHAPTER NINE
9.0 Beverages

9.1 Water

9.2 Herbal tea

9.3 Low-fat milk

9.4 Fruit juice

9.5 Lemon water

9.6 Homemade smoothies

9.7 Limit or avoid alcohol

CHAPTER TEN

10.0 Meal Planning

10.1 Establishing a Weekly Meal Plan

10.2 Grocery Shopping Tips

10.3 Planning Meals in Advance

10.4 CONCLUSION

CHAPTER ONE

1.0 Introduction

The kidneys play a key role in filtering waste and excess fluids from the body, and when they are not operating correctly, a tailored diet may help manage the symptoms and reduce the course of renal disease.

The major purpose of a renal diet is to restrict the quantity of protein, salt, potassium, and phosphorus in the diet. Protein is limited because it is broken down into waste products the kidneys must filter out. At the same time, salt, potassium, and phosphorus may build up in the circulation when the kidneys are not performing correctly.

A renal diet often comprises consuming foods low in sodium, potassium, and phosphorus and reducing the consumption of high-protein foods such as meat, dairy products, and eggs. Instead, persons with renal illness may be recommended to consume more fruits, vegetables, nutritious grains, and lean protein sources such as fish and poultry.

People with kidney disease must engage with their healthcare physician and a registered dietitian to design a tailored renal diet that matches their nutritional requirements and health objectives.

1.1 What is a Renal Diet?

A renal diet is a diet that is meant to manage and enhance the health of patients with kidney disease. The kidneys play a key role in filtering waste and excess fluid from the blood, and when they are not working correctly, it may lead to a buildup of toxins in the body. A renal diet aims to minimize the stress on the kidneys by restricting the consumption of specific nutrients that might be hazardous to those with kidney diseases, such as salt, potassium, phosphorus, and protein.

Some of the major components of a renal diet include:

- Reducing salt consumption could help manage blood pressure and prevent fluid retention

- Reducing potassium and phosphorus consumption to minimize the accumulation of these minerals in the blood, which may be hazardous to patients with renal disease

- Consuming a reasonable quantity of high-quality protein to assist in maintaining muscle mass while decreasing the stress on the kidneys

- Consuming lots of water to keep hydrated since dehydration may decrease kidney function

A renal diet is often recommended by a healthcare expert, such as a certified dietitian, who may recommend particular foods to consume or avoid and suggestions for meal planning and preparation.

1.2 Advantages of Following a Renal Diet

A renal diet is a specific meal plan aimed to assist patients with kidney disease manage their condition by minimizing the amount of waste and fluid in their bodies. The following are some of the advantages of adopting a renal diet:

1. **Improved kidney function:** A renal diet may help decrease the kidney's burden by decreasing the quantity of protein, salt, and potassium in the diet. This may slow down the course of renal disease and improve kidney function.

2. **Better blood pressure control:** A renal diet is often low in salt, which may help lower high blood pressure, a major consequence of kidney failure.

3. **Reduced risk of heart disease:** A renal diet may also help lessen the risk of heart disease, a major consequence of kidney illness. This is because the diet often reduces the consumption of saturated and trans fats, cholesterol, and processed carbohydrates.

4. **Improved overall health:** A renal diet may improve overall health by supporting good eating habits and avoiding other chronic illnesses such as diabetes and obesity.

5. **Better control of symptoms:** A renal diet may help manage symptoms such as fluid accumulation, nausea, and vomiting linked to kidney disease.

Adopting a renal diet may assist persons with kidney disease in managing their illness and enhance their quality of life.

Nonetheless, consulting a qualified dietitian is vital to establish a tailored renal diet that suits individual requirements and preferences.

1.3 How to Use This Cookbook

Utilizing a renal diet cookbook may be a terrific method to plan and prepare healthy meals for persons with kidney illnesses. Here are some recommendations for utilizing a renal diet cookbook:

1. **Read the introduction:** Start by reading the cookbook's introduction, which normally contains information about the renal diet, its advantages, and advice for following it.

2. **Search for meals that fit your demands:** Look for dishes that meet your dietary needs and tastes. For example, if you need to restrict your potassium consumption, seek dishes that are low in potassium. Similarly, if you are a vegetarian, seek meat-free dishes.

3. **Check the ingredients:** Before cooking, read the ingredients list to ensure they are compatible with a renal diet. If you need clarification about a specific component, contact a trained nutritionist.

4. **Pay attention to serving sizes:** The cookbook may give information on serving sizes and nutritional values for each dish. Attention to this information ensures you take only a little of any nutrient.

5. **Plan:** Utilize the cookbook to plan your meals for the week or month ahead. This may help you save time and minimize meal planning and preparation stress.

6. **Experiment:** Be bold and experiment with different recipes and ingredients. A renal diet cookbook may suggest tasty and healthy dishes that match your dietary demands.

Remember that a renal diet cookbook is a tool that may help you plan and prepare meals that are suited for your condition. Engaging with a qualified dietitian is crucial to design a tailored renal diet plan that suits your particular requirements and preferences.

CHAPTER TWO

2.0 Renal Diet Basics

A renal diet is a dietary strategy aimed at assisting persons with kidney disease to manage their illness and avoid additional kidney damage. The diet is often low in some nutrients, such as protein, salt, and potassium, and rich in others, such as fiber and vitamins.

The following are some essential elements of a renal diet:

1. **Limit protein intake:** Too much protein may increase the burden on the kidneys and lead them to perform less effectively. Your doctor or a qualified dietitian can assist decide

how much protein you should consume each day depending on your unique requirements.

2. **Control salt intake:** Sodium may promote fluid retention, burdening the kidneys. Reduce sodium consumption by avoiding processed meals, using herbs and spices instead of salt, and avoiding high-sodium condiments like soy sauce.

3. **Monitor potassium consumption:** Potassium is an important nutrient, but persons with renal illness may need to restrict their intake since their kidneys may be unable to eliminate excess potassium from the blood. Foods that are rich in potassium include bananas, potatoes, and tomatoes.

4. **Stay hydrated:** Consuming adequate water is vital to help keep the kidneys working correctly. Nevertheless,

persons with renal illness may need to restrict their fluid consumption if their kidneys cannot eliminate extra fluid from the body.

5. **Eat a balanced diet:** A diet rich in fruits, vegetables, whole grains, and lean meats will help you maintain a healthy weight and give your body the nutrients it needs.

Engaging with a qualified dietitian is crucial to design a tailored renal diet plan that suits your particular requirements and preferences.

2.1 Understanding Kidney Disease

Kidney disease, or renal disease, is when the kidneys are damaged and cannot operate effectively. The kidneys are two bean-shaped organs placed in the lower back, responsible for filtering waste materials and excess fluids from the blood, controlling blood pressure, and generating hormones that help manufacture red blood cells and keep bones strong.

There are numerous forms of kidney disease, including:

1. **Acute kidney injury (AKI):** A quick loss of kidney function caused by an abrupt reduction in blood supply to the kidneys, accident, or poisoning.

2. **Chronic kidney disease (CKD):** is a long-term disorder in which the kidneys progressively lose function. CKD may develop over many years and progress to end-stage kidney disease (ESKD) when the kidneys have lost practically all of their function.

3.   **Polycystic kidney disease (PKD):** A hereditary illness in which cysts grow in the kidneys and may lead to renal failure.

4.   **Glomerulonephritis:** A disorder in which the small filters in the kidneys become inflamed and damaged, which may lead to kidney failure.

Signs of kidney disease may only be obvious once the illness is advanced. Some typical symptoms include:

1. Fatigue

2. Swelling in the legs, ankles, feet, or face

3. Urinary changes, such as increased or reduced urination or black urine

4. Difficulty sleeping

5. Loss of appetite

6. Nausea and vomiting

7. Itching or dry skin

8. Muscle cramping

Therapy for kidney illness depends on the underlying cause and the degree of the condition. Possible treatments include drugs, adjustments to food and lifestyle, dialysis, or a kidney transplant. Engaging with a healthcare practitioner to treat renal illness and avoid complications is crucial.

2.2 Nutritional Needs for Renal Diets

Renal diets are dietary programs created for patients with renal disease, which may help control their illness and avoid complications.

Following are some of the important dietary needs for renal diets:

1. **Protein:** Individuals with renal illness may need to reduce their protein consumption since excessive protein may cause the kidneys to work harder. Yet, protein is still needed for sustaining muscle mass and general health. The quantity of protein required will depend on the severity of the renal disease and other individual characteristics.A nutritionist can assist in calculating the right quantity of protein for each individual.

2. **Sodium:** Too much sodium may cause the body to retain fluids, contributing to edema and high blood pressure. Individuals with renal illness may need to reduce their salt consumption, often to fewer than 2,300 milligrams daily. This may require avoiding processed foods and

restaurant meals, generally high in salt.

3. **Potassium:** The kidneys assist in controlling potassium levels in the body. If the kidneys are not working correctly, potassium levels may become excessively high, which can cause heart and muscle difficulties. Individuals with renal illness may need to reduce their potassium consumption, often to fewer than 2,000 mg daily. This may require avoiding high-potassium foods such as bananas, oranges, potatoes, and spinach.

4. **Phosphorus:** When the kidneys are not operating correctly, phosphorus levels may become excessively high, weakening bones and creating other health concerns. Individuals with renal illness may need to reduce their phosphorus consumption, often to

fewer than 1,000 mg daily. This may require avoiding high-phosphorus foods such as dairy products, nuts, and cola drinks.

5. **Fluids:** Individuals with renal disease may need to restrict their fluid consumption since the kidneys may be unable to eliminate excess fluid from the body. This may help avoid edema, high blood pressure, and other problems. The volume of fluid required will depend on the severity of the renal disease and other circumstances. A nutritionist can assist in determining the optimum quantity of hydration for each individual.

6. **Calories:** Individuals with kidney illness may need to alter their calorie intake, as significant weight gain or loss may burden the kidneys. The optimal calorie intake will depend on

the person's age, gender, weight, and activity level. A nutritionist may assist in calculating the optimal calorie intake for each individual.

The nutritional needs for renal diets may vary based on the person and the severity of the kidney disease. A certified dietitian can give specialized nutritional advice and assistance in building a meal plan that suits each person's particular requirements.

2.3 Foods to Limit or Avoid

Restricting or avoiding certain things in your diet would be best to preserve excellent health. Here are several examples:

1. **Processed Foods:** Meals that are heavily processed frequently include significant quantities of harmful fats, salt, and sugar. They may raise your

risk of heart disease, diabetes, and other chronic illnesses.

2. **Sugary Drinks:** Soda, sports, and energy drinks are rich in sugar and may contribute to weight gain and other health concerns.

3. **Fried Foods:** Fried meals like French fries, fried chicken, and doughnuts are heavy in calories and harmful fats. Consuming them often may raise your risk of heart disease, diabetes, and other chronic illnesses.

4. **Trans-Fats:** Trans fats are present in many processed meals, baked products, and fast food. These may boost your LDL (bad) cholesterol levels and increase your risk of heart disease.

5. **High-Sodium Foods:** Consuming too much salt may raise your blood

pressure and increase your heart disease and stroke risk. Avoid high-sodium meals such as canned soups, processed meats, and salty snacks.

6. **Refined Grains:** Refined grains like white bread, pasta, and rice have had their fiber and nutrients removed. They may trigger blood sugar increases and contribute to overeating.

7. **Alcohol:** Consuming too much alcohol may damage your liver and raise your chances of cancer, heart disease, and other health issues. It's preferable to minimize your consumption or avoid it completely.

Remember, moderation is crucial. It's good to indulge in these meals sometimes, but it's crucial to make healthy choices most of the time.

2.4 Items to Incorporate into a Renal Diet

A renal diet is meant to enhance kidney health and manage kidney illness. These are some things to include in a renal diet:

1. **Low-Potassium Fruits and Vegetables:** Fruits and vegetables are excellent sources of vitamins and minerals, but some are rich in potassium, which may be hazardous to persons with kidney disease. Excellent selections include apples, grapes, strawberries, cucumbers, and green beans.

2. **Low-Phosphorus Foods:** Excessive amounts of phosphorus in the blood

might harm the kidneys. Foods that are low in phosphorus include rice, pasta, bread, cauliflower, and egg whites.

3. **Lean Proteins:** Individuals with the renal illness must decrease their protein consumption but still require protein to maintain muscle mass. Excellent lean protein sources include chicken, turkey, fish, eggs, and tofu.

4. **Low-Sodium Foods:** Sodium may increase blood pressure and strain the kidneys. Look for low-sodium choices, including fresh veggies, unsalted almonds, and canned foods.

5. **Healthy Fats:** Although you should limit saturated and trans fats, healthy fats like olive oil, avocados, and almonds may deliver key nutrients and enhance heart health.

6. **Healthy Grains:** Whole grains like quinoa, brown rice, and whole wheat bread give fiber, vitamins, and minerals. They also have a lower glycemic index than refined grains, which may help manage blood sugar.

7. **Berries:** Berries are low in potassium and rich in antioxidants, making them a perfect option for persons with renal illness. Excellent selections include blueberries, raspberries, and strawberries.

Engaging with a healthcare expert and a registered dietitian is crucial to finding the appropriate renal diet for your unique kidney disease requirements and stage.

CHAPTER THREE

3.0 Morning Recipes

Renal breakfast dishes are meals created for those with renal disease who need to follow a particular diet to manage their illness. The kidneys are responsible for filtering waste and extra fluids from the body, but when they are not operating correctly, they may be unable to eliminate these substances adequately. A renal diet is meant to restrict the consumption of particular nutrients, such as sodium, phosphorus, and potassium, which may build up in the body and create difficulties.

Regarding renal breakfast dishes, it's vital to concentrate on meals low in sodium, phosphorus, and potassium while delivering appropriate nourishment.

3.1 oatmeal

3.1.1 Apple oatmeal custard:

Here's a recipe for Apple Oatmeal Custard:

Ingredients:

- 1 cup rolled oats
- 1 1/2 cups milk
- 1/4 teaspoon salt
- Two medium apples, peeled and sliced
- 1/4 cup brown sugar

- One teaspoon of ground cinnamon
- 1/4 teaspoon powdered nutmeg
- Two eggs
- One teaspoon of vanilla extract

Instructions:

1. Preheat the oven to 350°F.

2. Mix the rolled oats, milk, and salt in a medium-sized saucepan. Cook over medium heat, stirring periodically until the oatmeal is thick and creamy (approximately 10-12 minutes) (about 10-12 minutes).

3. Mix the cut apples, brown sugar, cinnamon, and nutmeg in a separate dish.

4. Grease a 9-inch baking dish with butter or cooking spray. Spoon the oats into the plate, then pour the apple mixture.

5. Mix the eggs and vanilla extract in a
    separate bowl. Pour the egg mixture
    over the cereal and apples.

6. Bake for 35-40 minutes until the top is
    golden brown and the custard has set.

7. Let cool for a few minutes before
    serving.

3.1.2 Strawberry and peanut oatmeal bowl

Here's a recipe for a Strawberry and Peanut
Oatmeal Bowl:

Ingredients:

- 1 cup rolled oats
- 2 cups water
- 1/4 teaspoon salt

- 1/4 cup chopped peanuts
- 1/4 cup sliced strawberries
- one tablespoon of honey
- 1/4 cup milk

Instructions:

1. In a medium-sized saucepan, bring the water to a boil. Add the oats and salt, then decrease the heat to medium-low. Simmer for approximately 5-7 minutes, stirring regularly, until the oatmeal is thick and creamy.

2. In a small pan, roast the chopped peanuts over medium heat for 2-3 minutes until nicely browned and aromatic.

3. Add the cut strawberries to the oatmeal and mix to incorporate.

4. Split the oatmeal into two dishes.
Drizzle each dish with honey and
sprinkle with the roasted peanuts.

5. Pour two teaspoons of milk over each
dish and serve immediately.

3.1.3 Blueberry overnight oats

Here's a recipe for Blueberry Overnight
Oats:

Ingredients:

- 1 cup rolled oats
- 1 cup milk (or non-dairy milk)
- 1/2 cup plain Greek yogurt
- 1 tablespoon honey (or maple syrup)
- 1/2 teaspoon vanilla extract
- 1/2 cup blueberries (fresh or frozen) (fresh or frozen)

Instructions:

1. Combine the rolled oats, milk, Greek yogurt, honey, and vanilla extract in a medium-sized mixing bowl. Mix thoroughly.

2. Fold in the blueberries and mix until equally distributed.

3. Cover the bowl with plastic wrap or a cover and refrigerate overnight (or at least 6-8 hours) (or at least 6-8 hours).

4. In the morning, toss the oats and add extra milk or yogurt if required to attain your preferred consistency.

5. Serve cold or reheat in the microwave for 1-2 minutes.

3.1.4 Strawberry chia overnight Oats

Here's a recipe for Strawberry Chia Overnight Oats:

Ingredients:

- 1 cup rolled oats
- 1 cup almond milk (or any other milk of your choice)
- 1/2 cup fresh strawberries, chopped
- 1 tablespoon chia seeds \s* 1 tablespoon honey (optional)
- 1/2 teaspoon vanilla extract
- Pinch of salt

Instructions:

1. In a large mixing bowl, combine the rolled oats, almond milk, sliced strawberries, chia seeds, honey (if using), vanilla essence, and a sprinkle

of salt. Stir everything together until fully blended.

2. Put the mixture into an airtight container like a mason jar. Cover and refrigerate overnight (or at least for 6-8 hours) (or 6-8 hours).

3. In the morning, give the mixture a thorough toss. If it's too thick, add more almond milk to thin it up to your preferred consistency.

4. Serve your Strawberry Chia, Overnight Oats, chilled, with more sliced strawberries on top if you prefer.

3.1.5 Strawberry chia overnight oats

Ingredients:

- 1/2 cup rolled oats

- 1/2 cup unsweetened almond milk (or any other milk of your choice)
- 1/2 cup sliced strawberries
- one tablespoon of chia seeds
- 1/2 teaspoon vanilla extract
- 1-2 tablespoons honey (optional)

Instructions:

1. In a bowl or mason jar, mix the rolled oats, almond milk, sliced strawberries, chia seeds, vanilla essence, and honey (if using) (if using).

2. Stir everything up until fully blended. Ensure the oats and chia seeds are well covered with the liquid.

3. Cover the dish or jar with a cover or plastic wrap and leave it in the refrigerator overnight (or for at least 4 hours) to let the oats and chia seeds soak and thicken.

4. In the morning, give the mixture a thorough toss. If it's too thick, add more almond milk to thin it up to your preferred consistency.

5. Serve your Strawberry Chia, Overnight Oats, chilled, with more sliced strawberries on top if you prefer.

3.1.6 Oatmeal porridge

Oatmeal porridge is a breakfast dish prepared from oats that have been cooked in water or milk. It is a popular and healthy morning item that is simple to cook and can be personalized with a variety of toppings and tastes.

To create oats porridge, you may start by boiling water or milk in a pot. Next, put in your oats and stir the mixture continually for around 5-10 minutes until the oats are cooked, and the mixture has thickened.

There are various types of oatmeal porridge, and you may add different toppings and flavorings to suit your preferences. Some common toppings include fresh fruit, nuts, honey, cinnamon, and brown sugar.

Oatmeal porridge is a nutritious breakfast choice since oats are abundant in fiber, protein, and vital elements like iron and magnesium. It is also a fantastic source of complex carbs, which give continuous energy throughout the morning.

3.2 Scrambled Eggs

3.2.1 Stuffed vegetable eggs

Ingredients:

- four big eggs
- 1/2 cup diced bell peppers
- 1/2 cup diced onions
- 1 cup chopped mushrooms
- 1 cup spinach leaves
- 1/2 cup diced tomatoes
- one tablespoon of olive oil
- Salt and pepper to taste
- **Optional:** shredded cheese, chopped herbs (such as parsley or chives)

Instructions:

1. Heat the olive oil over medium heat in a large pan.

2. Add the bell peppers, onions, and sauté for 2-3 minutes until softened.

3.   Add the mushrooms and continue to sauté for another 2-3 minutes until the mushrooms are cooked.

4.   Add the spinach leaves and toss until they are wilted.

5.   Add the chopped tomatoes and stir until they are cooked thoroughly.

6. Whisk the eggs with salt and pepper to taste in a separate dish.

7.   Pour the beaten eggs into the skillet with the veggies.

8.   Use a spatula to gently whisk the eggs and veggies together, cooking until the eggs are set to your preference.

9.   **Optional:** sprinkle with shredded cheese and chopped herbs before serving.

3.2.2 Scrambled eggs with kidney beans and cheddar

Ingredients:

- four eggs
- 1/2 cup of canned kidney beans, washed and rinsed
- 1/2 cup of shredded cheddar cheese
- 1 tablespoon of butter
- Salt & pepper to taste
- **Possible toppings:** chopped cilantro, spicy sauce, sliced avocado

Instructions:

1. Crack the eggs into a basin and whisk them together with a fork until fully beaten. Add salt and pepper to taste.

2.   Heat a large non-stick skillet over medium heat. Add the butter and let it melt.

3.   Once the butter has melted, add the kidney beans to the pan and simmer for 1-2 minutes, turning regularly, until they start to color slightly.

4.   Pour the eggs into the pan and let them cook for approximately 30 seconds until they start to set.

5.   Mix the eggs and beans together with a spatula until the eggs are scrambled and cooked through.

6.   Sprinkle the shredded cheddar cheese over the top of the eggs and beans and mix until the cheese is melted and evenly distributed.

7.   After thoroughly cooking the eggs, remove them from the fire and serve immediately with any preferred toppings.

Ingredients:

- four eggs
- 1/4 cup milk
- 1/4 cup diced red bell pepper
- 1/4 cup diced green bell pepper
- 1/4 cup diced onion
- 1/4 cup diced cooked ham
- 1/4 cup shredded cheddar cheese
- 2 tbsp butter
- Salt and pepper to taste

Instructions:

1. Crack the eggs into a bowl and mix with the milk—season with salt and pepper.

2. Melt the butter in a non-stick pan over medium-high heat.

3. Add the diced red and green bell peppers and onion to the pan and cook until they soften about 2-3 minutes.

4. Add the diced ham to the pan and cook for another 1-2 minutes.

5. Pour the egg mixture over the veggies and ham into the pan. Use a spatula to scramble the eggs, stirring regularly until they are cooked.

6. Sprinkle the shredded cheddar cheese over the top of the eggs and mix until melted.

7. Serve hot, and enjoy!

3.2.4 Tofu breakfast scramble

Ingredients:

- one block of firm tofu
- 1/2 tsp turmeric
- 1/2 tsp garlic powder
- 1/2 tsp onion powder
- Salt and pepper to taste
- 1 tbsp olive oil
- 1/4 cup diced onion
- 1/4 cup diced bell pepper
- 1/4 cup diced mushrooms
- 1/4 cup diced tomato
- 2 tbsp nutritional yeast (optional)
- Fresh parsley for garnish (optional)

Instructions:

1. Drain the tofu and wipe it dry with a paper towel. Use a fork to crush the tofu into tiny pieces.

2. Mix the turmeric, garlic powder, onion powder, salt, and pepper in a small bowl. Add this mixture to the crumbled tofu and stir until the tofu is coated.

3. Heat the olive oil in a non-stick pan over medium-high heat. Add the chopped onion, bell pepper, and mushrooms to the pan and sauté until they soften approximately 2-3 minutes.

4. Add the crushed tofu to the pan and simmer for 2-3 minutes, stirring regularly.

5. Add the diced tomato to the pan and simmer for 1-2 minutes.

6. If using, add the nutritional yeast to the pan and stir until mixed.

7. Serve hot and sprinkle with fresh parsley if preferred.

To make it your own, you may also personalize this dish by adding additional veggies such as spinach, kale, or zucchini.

3.2.5 Scrambled eggs, smashed avocado, and bean breakfast

Ingredients:

- two eggs

- 1/4 cup milk
- Salt and pepper, to taste
- 1 tbsp butter
- 1 avocado
- 1/2 lime
- 1/2 cup black beans, washed and rinsed
- 1/4 tsp cumin
- 1/4 tsp garlic powder
- 1/4 tsp chili powder
- 1 tbsp chopped cilantro

Instructions:

1. Crack the eggs into a bowl and add the milk, salt, and pepper. Mix until thoroughly blended.

2. Heat a non-stick pan over medium heat and add the butter. After the butter has melted, add the egg mixture.

3. Use a spatula to continually whisk the eggs until they are cooked to your desired consistency. Remove from heat and put aside.

4. Cut the avocado in half and remove the pit. Use a fork to mash the avocado in a bowl. Pour the lime juice over the avocado and season with salt and pepper.

5. In a separate skillet, cook the black beans over medium heat. Add the cumin, garlic, and chili powder, and mix until thoroughly incorporated.

6. To serve, lay the scrambled eggs on a platter and top them with the smashed avocado and black beans. Garnish with chopped cilantro. Enjoy your amazing scrambled eggs, smashed avocado, and bean breakfast!

3.3 smoothies

3.3.1 Blueberry blast smoothie

Ingredients:

- 1 cup frozen blueberries
- one frozen banana
- 1/2 cup plain Greek yogurt
- 1/2 cup almond milk (or any milk of your choice)
- 1 tablespoon honey (optional)

Instructions:

1. Add all the ingredients to a blender.

2. Blend on high speed for 1-2 minutes or until the mixture is smooth and creamy.

3. If the smoothie is too thick, add more milk until you achieve consistency.

4. Taste and adjust sweetness as required by adding additional honey.

5. Pour the smoothie into a glass and enjoy!

Optional Add-ins:

- one tablespoon of chia seeds
- 1 scoop of vanilla protein powder
- one tablespoon of almond butter
- 1/4 teaspoon cinnamon
- 1/2 teaspoon vanilla essence

3.3.2 Pineapple protein smoothie

Ingredients:

- 1 cup frozen pineapple chunks
- 1/2 banana
- one scoop of vanilla protein powder
- 1/2 cup plain Greek yogurt
- 1/2 cup unsweetened almond milk
- 1 teaspoon honey (optional)

Instructions:

1. Add the frozen pineapple chunks, banana, protein powder, Greek yogurt, almond milk, and honey (if using) to a blender.

2. Blend on high speed until smooth and creamy, approximately 30-60 seconds.

3. Pour the smoothie into a glass and enjoy!

You may modify the quantity of almond milk depending on how thick you prefer your smoothies. If you want a thinner smoothie, use more almond milk; if you want a thicker smoothie, use less. This smoothie is strong in protein, fiber, and vitamins, making it a nutritious and tasty breakfast alternative or post-workout snack.

3.3.3 Fruity smoothie

Ingredients:

- 1 cup frozen mixed berries (strawberries, blueberries, raspberries)
- one ripe banana
- 1/2 cup plain Greek yogurt
- 1/2 cup unsweetened almond milk \s*
  1 tablespoon honey (optional)

Instructions:

1. Add the frozen berries, banana, Greek yogurt, almond milk, and honey (if using) to a blender.

2. Blend on high speed until smooth and creamy.

3. Taste and adjust sweetness as required by adding additional honey.

4. Pour the smoothie into a glass and serve immediately.

3.3.4 Blended berry smoothie

Ingredients:

- 1 cup frozen mixed berries (strawberries, blueberries, raspberries)
- one ripe banana
- one scoop of vanilla protein powder
- 1/2 cup plain Greek yogurt
- 1/2 cup unsweetened almond milk
- 1 tablespoon honey (optional)

Instructions:

1. Add the frozen berries, banana, protein powder, Greek yogurt, almond milk, and honey (if using) to a blender.

2. Blend on high speed until smooth and creamy.

3. Taste and adjust sweetness as required by adding additional honey.

4. Pour the smoothie into a glass and serve immediately.

This smoothie is a terrific alternative for a post-workout snack or breakfast that will give you protein, fiber, and antioxidants to feed your body and keep you feeling full and content.

3.3.5 Peach High-Protein Smoothie

Ingredients:

- 1 ripe peach, peeled and sliced
- 1/2 cup plain Greek yogurt
- 1/2 cup unsweetened almond milk
- one scoop of vanilla protein powder
- one tablespoon of chia seeds
- 1/2 teaspoon vanilla extract
- 1-2 tablespoons honey (optional)

Instructions:

1. Add the sliced peach, Greek yogurt, almond milk, protein powder, chia seeds, vanilla extract, and honey (if using) to a blender.

2. Blend on high speed until smooth and creamy.

3. Taste and adjust sweetness as required by adding additional honey.

4. Pour the smoothie into a glass and serve immediately.

This peach high-protein smoothie is a delicious and healthy way to start your day or to refuel after a workout. Peaches are a great vitamin C and fiber source, while Greek yogurt and protein powder give protein to keep you full and content. The chia seeds offer beneficial fats and fiber, while the vanilla essence gives a wonderful taste.

3.3.6 Strawberry High-Protein Smoothie

Ingredients:

 1 cup frozen strawberries
To make it your own, you may also personalize this dish by adding additional veggies such as spinach, kale, or zucchini.

3.2.4 Scrambled eggs, smashed avocado, and bean breakfast

Ingredients:

* two eggs
* 1/4 cup milk

* Salt and pepper, to taste
* 1 tbsp butter
* 1 avocado
* 1/2 lime
* 1/2 cup black beans, washed and rinsed
* 1/4 tsp cumin
* 1/4 tsp garlic powder
* 1/4 tsp chili powder * 1 tbsp chopped cilantro

Instructions:

1. Crack the eggs into a bowl and add the milk, salt, and pepper. Mix until thoroughly blended.

2. Heat a non-stick pan over medium heat and add the butter. After the butter has melted, add the egg mixture.

3. Use a spatula to continually whisk the eggs until they are cooked to your desired consistency. Remove from heat and put aside.

4. Cut the avocado in half and remove the pit. Use a fork to mash the avocado in a bowl. Pour the lime juice over the avocado and season with salt and pepper.

5. In a separate skillet, cook the black beans over medium heat. Add the cumin, garlic, and chili powder, and mix until thoroughly incorporated.

6. To serve, lay the scrambled eggs on a platter and top them with the smashed avocado and black beans. Garnish with chopped cilantro. Enjoy your amazing scrambled eggs, smashed avocado, and bean breakfast!

3.4 Toast

3.4.1 Sprouted-grain toast with peanut butter and banana

Ingredients:

- 2 pieces of sprouted-grain bread \s* 2 tablespoons of natural peanut butter \s* 1 medium banana, sliced

Instructions:

1. Toast the sprouted-grain bread until it is golden brown.

2. Spread one tablespoon of natural peanut butter on each piece of bread.

3. Place the sliced banana on top of the peanut butter.

4. Serve and enjoy!

Sprouted-grain bread is a better alternative than ordinary bread because it is prepared from whole grains allowed to sprout, boosting their nutritional content and digestibility. Peanut butter is a great protein and healthy fats source, while bananas are rich in potassium, vitamins, and minerals. Together, they produce a substantial, refreshing meal that keeps you full and focused throughout the morning.

3.4.2 Whole grain peanut butter and fruit toast

Ingredients:

- 2 pieces of whole grain bread

- 2 tablespoons of natural peanut butter
- 1/2 cup of fresh fruit (such as sliced strawberries, blueberries, or bananas)
- **Optional:** honey, chia seeds, or sliced almonds for topping

Instructions:

1. Toast the whole grain bread until it is golden brown.

2. Spread one tablespoon of natural peanut butter on each piece of bread.

3. Arrange the cut fruit on top of the peanut butter.

4. Drizzle with honey, sprinkle with chia seeds, or add a few sliced almonds for taste and nutrition.

5. Serve and enjoy!

Whole-grain bread is a better alternative than white bread since it is created from whole grains high in fiber, vitamins, and minerals. Peanut butter is a wonderful source of protein and healthy fats, while fresh fruit delivers natural sweetness and a range of critical elements. This combination makes for a wonderful and gratifying breakfast or snack that will help keep you energetic and focused throughout the day.

3.4.3 Peanut butter and banana on toast

Peanut butter and banana on toast are traditional, tasty, and wholesome. Here's how to create it:

Ingredients:

- 1 ripe banana
- 2 pieces of bread

- 2-3 tablespoons of peanut butter
- Honey (optional) (optional)

Instructions:

1. Toast the bread to your chosen amount of crispiness.

2. Put peanut butter on both pieces of bread.

3. Peel the banana and cut it into thin slices.

4. Put the banana slices on one piece of bread.

5. Pour honey over the banana (optional) (optional).

6. Top the banana with the second piece of bread.

7.   Split the sandwich in half or into quarters, and enjoy!

You may also adjust this recipe by using almond butter or adding some cinnamon for added taste.

3.4.4 Peanut butter fruit toast

Ingredients:

- 2 pieces of whole wheat bread
- 2 tablespoons of peanut butter
- 1/2 banana, sliced
- 1/4 cup of fresh berries (such as strawberries, raspberries, or blueberries)
- 1 teaspoon of honey (optional)

Instructions:

1. Toast the pieces of bread until they are crispy.

2. Spread the peanut butter equally on both pieces of bread.

3. Place the sliced banana and fresh berries on the peanut butter.

4. Pour honey over the fruit, if preferred.

5. Serve and enjoy!

This recipe is flexible, so add or swap various fruits or nut jars of butter to your desire. You may also sprinkle chopped nuts or seeds for extra crunch and nutrients.

3.5 Bagel with Cream Cheese

3.5.1 Bagel with creamy cheese

Ingredients:

- 1 bagel, divided in half
- 2-3 tablespoons of creamy cheese (e.g., cream cheese, whipped cream cheese, flavored spreadable cheese)
- **Possible toppings:** sliced smoked salmon, cucumber, tomato, red onion, capers, fresh fruit, jam

Instructions:

1. Preheat your toaster or oven to your chosen amount of toasting.

2. Slice your Bagel in half and throw it in the toaster or oven.

3.   Toast the Bagel until it is golden brown and crispy outside.

4.   Once the Bagel is toasted, take it from the toaster or oven and set it on a plate or cutting board.

5.   Spread a substantial quantity of creamy cheese over each side of the Bagel. Use a knife or a spoon to distribute the cheese evenly.

6.   Place toppings on top of the cheese if you're using toppings. For example, you may add smoked salmon, cucumber slices, tomato slices, red onion, capers, fresh fruit, or jam.

7.   After you've added your favorite toppings, your Bagel with cream cheese is ready to enjoy!

3.5.2 Bagel with avocado and creamy cheese

Ingredients:

- one Bagel, sliced in half
- 1 ripe avocado, peeled and mashed
- 2-3 tablespoons of creamy cheese (e.g., cream cheese, whipped cream cheese, flavored spreadable cheese)
- Salt and pepper to taste
- **Optional toppings:** sliced tomatoes, sliced red onion, arugula, hot sauce

Instructions:

1. Preheat your toaster or oven to your desired level of toasting.

2. Split your Bagel in half and throw it in the toaster or oven.

3.   Toast the Bagel until it is golden brown and crispy outside.

4.   While the Bagel is toasting, prepare the avocado. Split the avocado in half, remove the pit, and scoop the flesh into a small dish. Mash the avocado with a fork until smooth, then add salt and pepper to taste.

5.   After the Bagel is cooked, take it from the toaster or oven and set it on a plate or cutting board.

6.   Put a substantial quantity of creamy cheese over each side of the Bagel. Use a knife or a spoon to distribute the cheese evenly.

7.   Put the mashed avocado on the cheese, distributing it equally between the two sides.

8. Place toppings on top of the avocado if you're using toppings. For example, add sliced tomatoes, red onion, arugula, or spicy sauce.

9. After you've added your favorite toppings, your Bagel with avocado and creamy cheese is ready to enjoy!

CHAPTER FOUR

4.0 Snack Recipes

Renal diet snack foods are meant to be kidney-friendly, meaning they are low in sodium, potassium, and phosphorus, which are nutrients that patients with the renal disease need to restrict.

4.1 Cranberry dip with fresh fruits

Ingredients:

- 1 cup fresh or frozen cranberries
- 1/4 cup honey
- 1 tbsp orange juice

- 1 tsp orange zest
- 8 oz cream cheese, softened
- Fresh fruit for dipping (such as apple slices, strawberries, or grapes).

Directions:

1. Mix the cranberries, honey, orange juice, and zest in a small saucepan. Simmer over medium heat, stirring periodically, until the cranberries burst and the sauce thickens slightly (approximately 10 minutes).

2. Remove the cranberry combination from the heat and allow it cool to room temperature.

3. In a separate bowl, whip the cream cheese until smooth and creamy.

4. Stir the chilled cranberry sauce into the cream cheese until completely mixed.

5. Chill the dip in the refrigerator for at least 30 minutes.

6. Serve the dip with fresh fruit for dipping.

Enjoy this tasty and kidney-friendly snack! Remember to speak to a certified dietitian if you have concerns about how this snack fits your overall nutritional requirements.

4.2 Tender ginger biscuits

Soft ginger cookies are a delightful and popular dessert that can be eaten any time of year, but they are especially popular in autumn and winter. Here's an easy recipe for creating soft ginger cookies:

Ingredients:

- 2 1/4 cups all-purpose flour
- 2 teaspoons ground ginger
- 1 teaspoon baking soda
- 3/4 teaspoon ground cinnamon
- 1/2 teaspoon ground cloves
- 1/4 teaspoon salt
- 3/4 cup unsalted butter, softened
- 1 cup granulated sugar
- 1 large egg
- 1/4 cup molasses
- 1/4 cup coarse sugar (for rolling cookies)

Instructions:

1. Preheat the oven to 350°F (175°C) and line a baking sheet with parchment paper.

2. Mix the flour, ginger, baking soda, cinnamon, cloves, and salt in a larger bowl.

3. Mix the butter and sugar together in a large basin until light and fluffy, approximately 2-3 minutes.

4. Add the egg and molasses to the butter mixture and whisk until thoroughly blended.

5. Add the dry ingredients to the wet components and stir until mixed.

6. Roll the dough into balls approximately one tablespoon in size, then coat each ball in coarse sugar.

7. Place the balls on the prepared baking sheet, allowing approximately 2 inches between them.

8. Bake for 10-12 minutes or until the sides are firm, but the centers are still soft.

9.   Allow the cookies to rest on the baking sheet for 5 minutes before cooling them on a wire rack.

10.   Serve and enjoy your lovely soft ginger cookies!

4.3 Delicious popcorn balls

Ingredients:

- 10 cups of popped popcorn
- 1 cup of sugar
- 1/2 cup of light corn syrup
- 1/2 cup of water
- 1/4 cup of butter
- 1/2 teaspoon of salt
- 1/2 teaspoon of vanilla essence

Instructions:

1. Preheat your oven to 250 degrees F.

2. Mix the sugar, corn syrup, water, butter, and salt in a large saucepan. Boil over medium heat, stirring regularly, until the mixture boils.

3. Once the mixture is boiling, stop stirring and let it simmer for another 5-7 minutes or until it reaches the hard ball stage (250-265 degrees F) on a candy thermometer.

4. Remove the saucepan from the heat and mix in the vanilla essence.

5. Pour the popped popcorn into a large mixing bowl and pour the hot sugar mixture over the top. Use a spatula to toss everything together until the popcorn is uniformly covered.

6. Let the mixture cool for a few minutes
    until it is cold enough to handle.

7. Grease your hands with cooking
    spray or butter and shape the dough
    into little balls.

8. Place the popcorn balls onto a baking
    sheet coated with parchment paper
    and bake for 20-25 minutes or until
    they are firm and slightly brown.

9. Let the popcorn balls cool fully before
    serving. You may preserve them in an
    airtight jar for up to a week.

4.4 Cucumber with sour cream

Ingredients:

- 1 big cucumber
- 1 cup sour cream
- 2 tablespoons minced fresh dill (optional)
- Salt and pepper to taste

Instructions:

1. Wash and peel the cucumber, Split it in half lengthwise and scoop out the seeds with a spoon, Chop the cucumber into tiny pieces.

2. Whisk together the sour cream and minced dill (if using) (if using).

3. Add the cucumber to the sour cream mixture and swirl well to incorporate.

4. Season with salt and pepper to taste.

5. Chill the cucumber and sour cream combination in the refrigerator for at least 30 minutes before serving to let the flavors melt together.

6. Serve as a dip with crackers, veggies, or topping for baked potatoes, grilled meats, or fish.

4.5 Hungarian sour cherry soup

Ingredients:

- 4 cups pitted sour cherries (fresh or frozen)
- 4 cups water
- 1 cinnamon stick
- 4-5 cloves

- 1/2 cup sugar (modify according to taste)
- 2 tablespoons cornstarch
- 1/2 cup sour \cream
- 1 teaspoon vanilla essence

Instructions:

1. Mix the cherries, water, cinnamon stick, and cloves in a large saucepan. Bring to a boil over medium heat, then drop the heat to low and simmer for 10-15 minutes.

2. Remove the cinnamon stick and cloves from the saucepan and discard.

3. Mix the sugar and cornstarch until completely incorporated in a separate bowl.

4. Add the sugar mixture to the saucepan with the cherries and stir

thoroughly. Cook for 5-10 minutes, stirring periodically until the soup has thickened somewhat.

5. Mix the sour cream and vanilla extract in a separate dish.

6. Remove the saucepan from the heat and whisk in the sour cream mixture until fully mixed.

7. Allow the soup to cool for a few minutes, then transfer to a blender and puree until smooth.

8. Chill the soup in the refrigerator for at least 2 hours before serving.

9. Serve the cooled soup in dishes or glasses, decorated with fresh mint leaves or whipped cream if preferred.

4.6 Sweet and sour meatballs

Ingredients:

4.6.1 For the meatballs:

- 1 pound shredded beef
- 1 egg
- 1/2 cup breadcrumbs
- 1/4 cup milk
- 1/4 cup chopped onion
- 1 tsp salt
- 1/2 tsp black pepper
- 1/4 tsp garlic powder

4.6.2 For the sweet and sour sauce:

- 1/2 cup ketchup
- 1/4 cup white vinegar
- 1/4 cup brown sugar

- 2 tbsp soy sauce
- 1 tbsp cornstarch
- 1/4 cup water
- 1/2 cup pineapple chunks

Instructions:

1. Preheat the oven to 400°F.

2. Combine the ground beef, egg, breadcrumbs, milk, chopped onion, salt, black pepper, and garlic powder in a large mixing bowl. Stir thoroughly until all components are properly incorporated.

3. Using your hands, shape the mixture into 1-inch meatballs and lay them on a baking sheet.

4. Bake the meatballs in the preheated oven for 15-20 minutes, or until they are thoroughly cooked.

5. Make the sweet and sour sauce while the meatballs are baking. Mix the ketchup, white vinegar, brown sugar, soy sauce, and pineapple pieces in a medium saucepan. Bring the mixture to a boil over medium-high heat, stirring frequently.

6. Mix the cornstarch and water in a small bowl until the cornstarch is thoroughly dissolved.

7. Once the sauce is bubbling, decrease the heat to medium-low and gently whisk in the cornstarch mixture. Continue to whisk the sauce until it thickens, which should take approximately 1-2 minutes.

8. Once the meatballs are done, take them from the oven and transfer them to a large mixing dish.

9.   Pour the sweet and sour sauce over the meatballs and gently toss them until the sauce is equally distributed.

10.   Serve the sweet and sour meatballs hot, topped with more pineapple pieces or chopped scallions, if preferred.

4.7 Hot cornbread

Ingredients:

- 1 cup yellow cornmeal
- 1 cup all-purpose flour
- 1/4 cup sugar
- 1 tbsp baking powder
- 1 tsp salt
- 1/4 tsp cayenne pepper

- 1/4 tsp chili powder
- 1/4 cup chopped jalapeño peppers
- 1/2 cup shredded cheddar cheese \s*
  2 eggs
- 1 cup milk
- 1/4 cup vegetable oil

Instructions:

1. Preheat the oven to 400°F.

2. Add the cornmeal, flour, sugar, baking powder, salt, cayenne pepper, and chili powder in a large mixing bowl. Stir thoroughly until all dry ingredients are properly mixed.

3. Stir in the chopped jalapeño peppers and grated cheddar cheese.

4. Whisk the eggs, milk, and vegetable oil in a separate mixing bowl until smooth.

5. Pour the wet components into the dry ingredients and whisk until incorporated. Do not overmix the batter.

6. Pour the batter into a prepared 9-inch square baking dish.

7. Bake the cornbread in the oven for 20-25 minutes or until a toothpick inserted into the middle comes out clean.

8. After the cornbread, take it from the oven and allow it to cool for 5-10 minutes before slicing and serving.

4.8 Hot crunchy and munch snack combo

If you're searching for a delicious and spicy snack mix that's excellent for parties, movie nights, or whenever you need a crunchy snack, try preparing this recipe for spicy crunchy, and munch snack mix:

Ingredients:

- 2 cups Chex cereal (your choice of flavor)
- 2 cups pretzel sticks
- 1 cup roasted salted peanuts
- 1/2 cup butter
- 1 tbsp Worcestershire sauce
- 2 tsp hot sauce
- 1 tsp garlic powder
- 1 tsp onion powder
- 1 tsp chili powder
- 1/4 tsp cayenne pepper

Instructions:

1. Preheat the oven to 250°F.

2. Add the Chex cereal, pretzel sticks, and toasted peanuts to a large mixing bowl.

3. Melt the butter in a small saucepan over medium heat.

4. Once the butter is melted, whisk in the Worcestershire sauce, hot sauce, garlic powder, onion powder, chili powder, and cayenne pepper. Stir thoroughly until all components are properly incorporated.

5. Pour the spicy butter sauce over the snack mix in the mixing bowl and whisk until all ingredients are uniformly covered.

6. Spread the snack mix in a single layer on a large baking sheet.

7. Bake the snack mix in the preheated oven for 1 hour, stirring every 15 minutes.

. After the snack mix is done, take it from the oven and allow it to cool fully before serving.

4.9 Sweet and spicy tortilla chips

Ingredients:

- 8-10 corn tortillas
- 1/4 cup vegetable oil
- 2 tbsp honey
- 1 tbsp brown sugar
- 1 tsp chili powder
- 1/2 tsp paprika

- 1/4 tsp cumin
- 1/4 tsp garlic powder
- 1/4 tsp salt

Instructions:

1. Preheat the oven to 350°F.

2. Cut the tortillas into tiny triangles and place them in a single layer on a baking sheet.

3. Mix the vegetable oil, honey, brown sugar, chili powder, paprika, cumin, garlic powder, and salt in a separate bowl.

4. Brush the mixture evenly over the tortilla triangles.

5. Bake the tortillas in the oven for 10-12 minutes or until crispy and golden brown.

6. Remove the tortillas from the oven and allow them to cool for a few minutes.

7. Serve the sweet and spicy tortilla chips with your favorite salsa or dip.

4.10 Addictive pretzels

Ingredients:

- 1 lb. of pretzel twists or sticks
- 1/2 cup vegetable oil
- 1/4 cup Worcestershire sauce
- 1/4 cup soy sauce
- 1 tbsp garlic powder
- 1 tsp onion powder
- 1 tsp dried oregano
- 1 tsp dried basil

Instructions:

1. Preheat the oven to 250°F.

2. Whisk together the vegetable oil, Worcestershire sauce, soy sauce, garlic powder, onion powder, oregano, and basil in a large mixing bowl.

3. Add the pretzels to the mixing bowl and toss them in the sauce until they are equally covered.

4. Arrange the pretzels in a single layer on a baking sheet coated with parchment paper.

5. Bake the pretzels in the oven for 1 hour, tossing every 15-20 minutes to achieve equal cooking.

6. After an hour, take the pretzels from the oven and allow them to cool for a few minutes.

7. Offer the addicting pretzels as a snack or party starter.

4.11 Shrimp spray with crackers

Ingredients:

- 1 pound cooked shrimp, peeled and deveined
- 8 oz cream cheese, softened
- 1/4 cup mayonnaise
- 1/4 cup sour cream
- 2 cloves garlic, minced
- 1 tbsp lemon juice
- 1 tsp Worcestershire sauce
- 1/2 tsp salt
- 1/4 tsp black pepper
- 1/4 cup chopped fresh parsley

- Crackers for serving

Instructions:

1. In a food processor, pulse the cooked shrimp until finely minced.

2. Add the cream cheese, mayonnaise, sour cream, garlic, lemon juice, Worcestershire sauce, salt, and pepper to the food processor.

3. Pulse the mixture until it is smooth and fully blended.

4. Transfer the shrimp spread to a serving dish and toss in the chopped parsley.

5. Serve the shrimp spread with your favorite crackers.

4.12 Wonton quiche minis

Ingredients:

- 24 wonton wrappers
- 4 eggs \s* 1/2 cup milk
- 1/2 cup shredded cheddar cheese
- 1/2 cup diced ham
- 1/4 cup diced red bell pepper
- 1/4 cup chopped green onions
- Salt and pepper, to taste

Instructions:

1. Preheat the oven to 375°F.

2. Spray a muffin pan with cooking spray.

3. Carefully press a wonton wrapper into each muffin cup, carefully pushing the wrapper down and into the corners of the cup.

4. Whisk the eggs and milk until thoroughly blended in a medium mixing basin.

5. Add the shredded cheese, diced ham, diced red bell pepper, chopped green onions, salt, and pepper to the mixing bowl and toss until thoroughly blended.

6. Spoon the egg mixture into the wonton cups, filling each cup approximately 3/4 of the way full.

7. Bake the wonton quiche minis in the oven for 15-18 minutes, until the eggs are set and the wonton wrappers are golden brown.

8. Remove the wonton quiche minis from the oven and let them cool in the muffin tray for a few minutes.

9. Carefully remove the wonton quiche
    minis from the muffin tray and serve
    them warm.

CHAPTER FIVE

5.0   Salad   and   Appetizer Recipes

Renal salads and appetizers are foods that are particularly prepared to fulfill the dietary limitations and nutritional demands of patients with renal (kidney) illnesses. Individuals with renal illness typically have to follow a particular diet to avoid additional kidney damage and manage their symptoms.

Renal salads and appetizers often contain items that are low in sodium, potassium, and phosphorus, while still delivering critical nutrients like protein, fiber, and vitamins. They are also intended to be delicious and fulfilling so that persons with renal illness may enjoy a diverse and balanced diet.

5.1 Cool coconut marshmallow salad

Ingredients:

- 1 (20 oz) can crush pineapple, drained
- 1 (3.4 oz) packet instant vanilla pudding mix
- 1 cup small marshmallows
- 1 cup shredded coconut
- 1 cup whipped cream or whipped topping
- Maraschino cherries, for garnish (optional)

Instructions:

1. Combine the drained crushed pineapple and instant vanilla pudding mix in a large mixing dish.

2. Mix in the tiny marshmallows and crushed coconut until fully blended.

3. Stir in the whipped cream or topping until the mixture is smooth and creamy.

4. Cover the bowl with plastic wrap and refrigerate for at least 1 hour or until the salad has cooled and firm.

5. After cooling, give the salad a brief swirl to ensure all ingredients are uniformly distributed.

6. If preferred, serve the chilled coconut marshmallow salad in separate dishes or cups, topped with maraschino cherries.

5.2 Pineapple coleslaw

Ingredients:

- 1 (20 oz) can crush pineapple, drained
- 1 (3.4 oz) packet instant vanilla pudding mix

- 1 cup small marshmallows
- 1 cup shredded coconut
- 1 cup whipped cream or whipped topping
- Maraschino cherries, for garnish (optional)

Instructions:

1. Combine the drained crushed pineapple and instant vanilla pudding mix in a large mixing dish.

2. Stir in the tiny marshmallows and crushed coconut until fully blended.

3. Fold in the whipped cream or topping until the mixture is smooth and creamy.

4. Cover the bowl with plastic wrap and refrigerate for at least 1 hour or until the salad has cooled and firm.

5. Once cooled, give the salad a brief swirl to ensure all ingredients are uniformly distributed.

6. If preferred, serve the chilled coconut marshmallow salad in separate dishes or cups, topped with maraschino cherries.

5.3 Pineapple coleslaw

Ingredients:

- 1 (16 oz) bag coleslaw mix (shredded cabbage and carrots)
- 1 cup diced fresh pineapple
- 1/4 cup diced red onion
- 1/4 cup chopped fresh cilantro
- 1/4 cup mayonnaise
- 1/4 cup plain Greek yogurt
- 2 teaspoons apple cider vinegar
- 2 tablespoons honey
- Salt and black pepper, to taste

Instructions:

1. Combine the coleslaw mix, diced pineapple, red onion, and chopped cilantro in a large mixing bowl.

2. In a separate bowl, mix the mayonnaise, Greek yogurt, apple

cider Vinegar, honey, salt, and black pepper until smooth and thoroughly incorporated.

3. Pour the dressing over the coleslaw mixture and toss until everything is equally covered.

4. Cover the bowl with plastic wrap and refrigerate for at least 1 hour or until the coleslaw is cooled and the flavors have blended.

5. Once cooled, give the coleslaw a brief swirl to ensure all ingredients are uniformly distributed.

6. Serve the pineapple coleslaw as a side dish or on top of grilled burgers or sandwiches.

5.4 Low-salt macaroni and cheese

Ingredients:

- 8 ounces elbow macaroni
- 2 tablespoons unsalted butter
- 2 tablespoons all-purpose flour
- 2 cups low-sodium milk
- 1/4 teaspoon garlic powder
- 1/4 teaspoon black pepper
- 1/4 teaspoon dry mustard
- 2 cups shredded low-sodium cheddar cheese
- 1/4 cup breadcrumbs

Instructions:

1. Preheat the oven to 350°F (175°C) and gently butter a 9-inch baking dish.

2. Cook the macaroni according to package directions until al dente. Drain and put aside.

3. In a medium saucepan, melt the butter over medium heat.

4. Whisk in the flour and cook for 1-2 minutes, stirring frequently, until the mixture is smooth and bubbling.

5. Gradually mix the milk, garlic powder, black pepper, and dry mustard. Simmer, stirring frequently, until the mixture boils and thickens, approximately 5-7 minutes.

6. Remove the skillet from the heat and whisk the shredded cheddar cheese until thoroughly blended.

7. Add the cooked macaroni to the cheese sauce and mix until evenly covered.

8. Transfer the macaroni and cheese mixture to the prepared baking dish and sprinkle the breadcrumbs on top.

9.   Bake for 20-25 minutes until the breadcrumbs are golden brown and the cheese is bubbling.

10.   Remove the dish from the oven and allow it to cool for a few minutes before serving.

5.5 Low-salt macaroni and cheese

Ingredients:

- 8 ounces elbow macaroni
- 1 tablespoon unsalted butter
- 1 tablespoon all-purpose flour
- 1 cup low-fat milk
- 1 cup shredded reduced-fat cheddar cheese
- 1/4 teaspoon black pepper
- 1/4 teaspoon paprika

Directions:

1. Cook macaroni according to package directions. Drain and put aside.
2. In a saucepan, melt butter over medium heat. Add flour and mix until smooth.

3. Gradually add milk, frequently stirring, until the mixture is smooth.

4. Bring mixture to a boil and simmer for 1-2 minutes or until it thickens.

5. Reduce heat to low and whisk in shredded cheddar cheese until melted.

6. Add black pepper and paprika and mix until blended.

7. Add cooked macaroni to cheese sauce and toss until macaroni is covered with sauce.

8. Serve hot.

Note: If you want a lower-fat option, you may swap the reduced-fat cheddar cheese with a low-fat or fat-free cheese alternative. Moreover, you may add veggies such as broccoli or cauliflower to the mix for extra nourishment.

5.6 Buffalo chicken salad cucumber cups

Ingredients:

- 1/2 cup cooked and shredded chicken breast
- 1/4 cup buffalo sauce
- 1/4 cup plain Greek yogurt
- 2 tablespoons crumbled blue cheese
- 2 cucumbers
- Salt and pepper to taste
- **Optional garnish:** chopped fresh parsley or green onions

Instructions:

1. Mix the shredded chicken, buffalo sauce, Greek yogurt, and crumbled blue cheese in a medium bowl until thoroughly blended.

2. Season with salt and pepper to taste.

3. Using a vegetable peeler, peel off strips of the cucumber skin lengthwise, leaving some skin on to form a striped pattern.

4. Cut the cucumbers into thick circles, approximately 1 1/2 inches thick.

5. Use a small spoon or a melon baller to scoop out the center of each cucumber round, leaving approximately 1/4 inch of cucumber flesh around the edge to make a cup.

6. Spoon a tiny quantity of the buffalo chicken salad into each cucumber cup.

7. Garnish with chopped fresh parsley or green onions, if preferred.

8. Serve immediately or chill in the refrigerator until ready to serve.

5.7 Chili cornbread casserole

Ingredients:

For the chili

- 1 pound of beef
- 1 onion, chopped
- 1 bell pepper, chopped
- 2 cloves garlic, minced
- 1 can (14.5 ounces) diced tomatoes
- 1 can (15 ounces) kidney beans, drained and rinsed
- 1 tablespoon chili powder

- 1 teaspoon cumin
- Salt and pepper to taste

For the cornmeal topping:

- 1 cup cornmeal
- 1 cup all-purpose flour
- 1/4 cup granulated sugar
- 1 tablespoon baking powder
- 1/2 teaspoon salt
- 1 cup milk
- 1/4 cup vegetable oil
- 1 egg

Instructions:

1. Preheat the oven to 400°F (200°C).

2. In a large pan, cook the ground beef over medium-high heat.

3. Add the onion, bell pepper, and garlic to the pan and sauté until the veggies are soft, approximately 5 minutes.

4. Add the chopped tomatoes (with their liquid), kidney beans, chili powder, cumin, salt, and pepper to the pan. Bring the mixture to a simmer and cook for 10 minutes.

5. Pour the chili into a 9x13-inch baking dish.

6. Mix the cornmeal, flour, sugar, baking powder, and salt in a separate basin.

7. Mix the milk, vegetable oil, and egg in another dish.

8. Add the wet and dry ingredients to whisk until just blended.

9. Pour the cornbread batter over the chili in the baking dish.

10. Bake for 25-30 minutes until the cornbread is golden brown and a

toothpick inserted into the middle comes out clean.

11.   Let the dish cool for a few minutes before serving.

5.8 Caribbean lime shrimp salad

Ingredients:

For the salad:

- 1 pound cooked shrimp, peeled and deveined
- 1 mango, peeled and diced
- 1 avocado, peeled and diced
- 1/2 red onion, diced
- 1/4 cup chopped fresh cilantro

For the dressing:

- 1/4 cup lime juice
- 1/4 cup olive oil
- 1 tablespoon honey

- 1 tablespoon Dijon mustard
- 1/2 teaspoon salt
- 1/4 teaspoon black pepper

Instructions:

1. Add the cooked shrimp, diced mango, avocado, red onion, and chopped cilantro in a large bowl.

2. Mix the lime juice, olive oil, honey, Dijon mustard, salt, and black pepper in a separate bowl.

3. Pour the dressing over the salad and toss to coat.

4. Serve immediately, topped with more cilantro if desired.

5.9 Creamy caesar salad-keto renal

Ingredients:

For the salad:

- 1 head of Romaine lettuce, chopped
- 1 can (15 ounces) kidney beans, drained and rinsed
- 1/4 cup grated Parmesan cheese
- Salt & pepper to taste

For the dressing:

- 1/4 cup mayonnaise
- 1/4 cup grated Parmesan cheese
- 2 teaspoons fresh lemon juice
- 1 tablespoon Dijon mustard \s* 1 clove garlic, minced
- Salt and pepper to taste
- 1/4 cup olive oil

Instructions:

1. Mix the chopped Romaine lettuce and kidney beans in a large dish.

2. Add the shredded Parmesan cheese, salt, and pepper to the bowl.

3. Mix the mayonnaise, grated Parmesan cheese, fresh lemon juice, Dijon mustard, chopped garlic, salt, and pepper in a separate dish.

4. Slowly whisk in the olive oil until the dressing is completely blended.

5. Drizzle the dressing over the salad and toss to coat.

6. Serve immediately, topped with more Parmesan cheese if preferred.

5.10 Blackberry spinach salad

Ingredients:

- 4 cups baby spinach
- 1 cup blackberries

- 1/4 cup sliced almonds
- 1/4 cup crumbled feta cheese
- 2 teaspoons balsamic vinegar
- 2 tablespoons olive oil
- 1 tablespoon honey
- Salt and pepper to taste

Instructions:

1. Mix the baby spinach, blackberries, sliced almonds, and crumbled feta cheese in a large bowl.

2. Mix the balsamic vinegar, olive oil, honey, salt, and pepper in a separate dish.

3. Drizzle the dressing over the salad and toss to coat.

4. Serve immediately, topped with more sliced almonds and blackberries if preferred.

CHAPTER SIX

6.0 Main Dish Recipes

Renal main dishes are meals tailored to fulfill the dietary limitations and nutritional demands of patients with renal (kidney) illnesses. Individuals with renal illness typically have to follow a particular diet to avoid additional kidney damage and manage their symptoms.

Renal main courses often comprise lean protein sources, minimal levels of sodium, and restricted amounts of potassium, phosphorus, and other minerals. The meals are also meant to be savory and enjoyable so that persons with renal illness may enjoy a diverse and nutritious diet.

Some examples of main renal courses are grilled chicken with roasted vegetables, baked salmon with steaming green beans, and lentil soup with a side salad. These recipes are cooked using foods low in sodium, potassium, and phosphorus while delivering key nutrients like protein, fiber, and vitamins.

It's vital to check with a healthcare practitioner or certified dietitian before making any dietary changes, particularly if you have a renal illness. They may provide specialized assistance and meal plans for your unique requirements and objectives.

6.1 Grain hot cereal

Ingredients:

- 1/2 cup steel-cut oats
- 1/2 cup quinoa
- 1/2 cup amaranth

- 3 cups water
- 1/4 tsp salt
- 1/4 cup milk
- 1/4 cup chopped nuts (optional)
- 1/4 cup dried fruit (optional)
- Honey or maple syrup to taste (optional)

Instructions:

1. Rinse the quinoa and amaranth well under running water.

2. Mix the steel-cut oats, quinoa, amaranth, water, and salt in a medium-sized saucepan.

3. Bring the mixture to a boil over high heat, then decrease the heat to medium and let simmer for 20-25 minutes, stirring periodically.

4. Remove the saucepan from heat once the grains are soft and the water has been absorbed.

5. Stir in the milk, chopped almonds, dried fruit, and honey or maple syrup (if using) (if using).

6. Cover the pot and let the mixture rest for 5 minutes to enable the flavors to mingle.

7. Divide the wild cereal into dishes and serve immediately, topped with more nuts and fruit if preferred.

Note: This recipe yields around four servings but may easily be doubled or reduced depending on your requirements. You may also alter the recipe by adding your favorite spices, such as cinnamon or nutmeg, or using various kinds of milk, such as almond or soy.

6.2 Baba ghanoush

Ingredients:

- 2 medium eggplants
- 1/4 cup tahini
- 2 garlic cloves, minced
- 1/4 cup fresh lemon juice
- 1/4 cup olive oil
- 1/4 tsp ground cumin
- Salt and pepper to taste
- Chopped fresh parsley for garnish

Instructions:

1. Preheat the oven to 400°F.

2. Cut the eggplants in half lengthwise and set them cut-side down on a baking pan.

3. Roast the eggplants in the oven for 30-35 minutes or until extremely tender.

4. Let the eggplants cool, then scoop out the meat and discard the skins.

5. Mix the eggplant meat, tahini, garlic, lemon juice, olive oil, cumin, salt, and pepper in a food processor or blender.

6. Process the ingredients until smooth and creamy.

7. Taste and adjust the seasoning as required.

8. Transfer the baba ghanoush to a serving dish and top with chopped fresh parsley.

9. Serve with pita bread or fresh veggies for dipping.

Note: You may grill the eggplants instead of roasting them for a smokier taste. Just spray the eggplant halves with olive oil and grill them over medium-high heat until they are blackened and extremely tender, approximately 10-15 minutes on each side.

6.3 Beef and vegetable kebabs

Ingredients:

- 1 lb beef sirloin, cut into 1-inch cubes
- 2 bell peppers, cut into 1-inch pieces
- 1 red onion, cut into 1-inch pieces
- 8-10 cherry tomatoes
- 1/4 cup olive oil
- 2 garlic cloves, minced
- 2 tbsp fresh lemon juice
- 1 tsp ground cumin
- 1 tsp smoky paprika
- Salt and pepper to taste

- Wooden skewers, soaking in water for 30 minutes

Instructions:

1. Preheat the grill to medium-high heat.

2. Mix the olive oil, garlic, lemon juice, cumin, smoked paprika, salt, and pepper in a large bowl.

3. Add the meat cubes to the bowl and mix to coat with the marinade. Let the beef marinade for at least 30 minutes or up to 2 hours.

4. Thread the marinated meat, bell peppers, red onion, and cherry tomatoes onto the wet wooden skewers, rotating the ingredients as you go.

5. Grill the kebabs for 8-10 minutes, rotating regularly, or until the meat is cooked to your satisfaction and the veggies are soft and gently browned.

6. Remove the kebabs from the grill and let them rest for a few minutes before serving.

Note: You may personalize this dish by adding other kinds of veggies or meat. You may add some spice to the marinade by adding chili flakes or using hotter paprika.

6.4 Broccoli, garlic, and rigatoni

Ingredients:

- 1 lb rigatoni pasta

- 1 head broccoli, chopped into tiny florets
- 4 garlic cloves, minced
- 1/4 cup olive oil
- Salt and pepper to taste
- Grated Parmesan cheese for serving (optional)

Instructions:

1. Cook the rigatoni pasta in a large pot of salted boiling water according to the package directions until al dente.

2. Heat the olive oil in a large pan over medium heat while the pasta is boiling.

3. Add the minced garlic to the pan and heat for 1-2 minutes or until fragrant and gently brown.

4. Add the broccoli florets to the pan and swirl to coat with the garlic and

oil—season with salt and pepper to taste.

5. Cook the broccoli for 5-7 minutes, occasionally stirring until tender and lightly browned.

6. Once the pasta is done, rinse it and return it to the pan with broccoli and garlic.

7. Toss everything together to mix, adding a splash of pasta water if required to loosen the sauce.

8. Serve the pasta hot, topped with grated Parmesan cheese if preferred.

Note: You may add some spice to the meal by adding red pepper flakes to the garlic and oil combination. You may also replace different kinds of pasta or veggies, such as cauliflower or asparagus, to make the recipe your own.

6.5 Chicken brats

Chicken brats are a sausage prepared with ground chicken flesh and different spices. They are often cooked with a blend of chicken meat, spices, and herbs and may contain additional items like vegetables, cheese, or fruit. Chicken brats may be prepared in several methods, including grilling, baking, or pan-frying, and are commonly served with toppings and sauces.

They are a popular alternative to regular pig bratwurst for people who want a leaner meat choice or who avoid pork for religious or nutritional reasons.

6.6 Chicken salad with pineapple balsamic vinaigrette

Ingredients for Chicken Salad:

- 2 cups cooked chicken, shredded or cubed
- 1 cup chopped celery
- 1 cup diced pineapple
- 1/4 cup chopped red onion
- 1/4 cup chopped fresh parsley
- Salt and pepper to taste

Ingredients for Pineapple Balsamic Vinaigrette:

- 1/2 cup fresh pineapple chunks
- 1/4 cup balsamic vinegar
- 1/4 cup extra-virgin olive oil
- 1 tablespoon honey
- Salt and pepper to taste

Instructions:

1. In a large dish, mix the cooked chicken, chopped celery, cubed pineapple,

2. Mix the pineapple chunks, balsamic vinegar, olive oil, honey, salt, and pepper until smooth in a blender or food processor.

3. Pour the pineapple balsamic vinaigrette over the chicken salad and toss to coat.

4. Serve immediately or chill in the refrigerator until ready to serve.

6.7 Corn tamales with avocado-tomatillo salsa

Ingredients for Corn Tamales:

- 2 cups masa harina
- 1 teaspoon baking powder
- 1 teaspoon salt
- 1 1/2 cups vegetable broth
- 1/2 cup vegetable shortening
- 2 cups fresh corn kernels
- Corn husks, steeped in water for at least 2 hours

Ingredients for Avocado-Tomatillo Salsa:

- 2 medium tomatillos, husks removed and washed
- 1 avocado, pitted and diced
- 1/2 red onion, diced
- 1 garlic clove, minced
- 1/4 cup fresh cilantro leaves

- Juice of 1 lime \s* Salt and pepper to taste

Instructions:

1. Combine the masa harina, baking powder, and salt in a large mixing basin. Add the veggie broth and shortening and stir until fully blended.

2. Mix the fresh corn kernels in a food processor until they form a thick paste. Add the corn to the masa mixture and stir thoroughly.

3. Take a corn husk and apply a thin layer of masa mixture over the middle of the husk, leaving approximately an inch of space on the edges. Flip the husk over and wrap it up securely. Continue until all the masa mixture is used up.

4. Place the tamales in a steamer basket and steam for approximately 1 hour or until the masa is firm and cooked thoroughly.

5. While the tamales are heating, create the avocado-tomatillo salsa. In a blender or food processor, puree the tomatillos, avocado, red onion, garlic, cilantro, lime juice, salt, and pepper until smooth.

6. Serve the heated tamales with the avocado-tomatillo salsa on top. Enjoy your wonderful Corn Tamales with Avocado-Tomatillo Salsa!

6.8 Fettuccine with clams, brazil, tomato, corn, and garlic

Ingredients:

- 1 pound fettuccine pasta
- 2 dozen fresh clams, cleaned clean
- 3 tablespoons olive oil
- 4 cloves garlic, minced
- 1 can of corn (or 1 cup of fresh corn kernels)
- 2 tomatoes, diced
- 1/4 cup white wine
- 1/4 cup chopped fresh parsley
- Salt and pepper to taste

Instructions:

1. Cook the fettuccine pasta in a large pot of salted boiling water until al dente, following the package

directions. Rinse the pasta and keep it aside.

2. Heat the olive oil over medium heat in a large pan. Add the minced garlic and sauté for 1-2 minutes or until fragrant.

3. Add the diced tomatoes and corn to the pan, and sauté for another 2-3 minutes or until the tomatoes are tender.

4. Pour in the white wine and bring the mixture to a boil.

5. Add the clams to the pan, and cover with a lid. Cook for 5-7 minutes or until the clams open up. Discard any clams that do not open.

6. Add the cooked fettuccine pasta to the pan, and combine with the clam and tomato sauce.

7. Season with salt and pepper to taste, then sprinkle with chopped fresh parsley.

8. Serve the fettuccine with clams, Brazil, tomato, corn, and garlic hot, and enjoy!

6.9 Fish tacos with tomatillo sauce

Ingredients:

- 1 pound white fish (such as tilapia or cod)
- 1 teaspoon chili powder
- 1 teaspoon cumin
- 1/2 teaspoon paprika
- Salt and pepper to taste
- 2 tablespoons olive oil
- 8 corn tortillas
- 1 cup shredded cabbage

- 1/4 cup chopped fresh cilantro
- 1 lime, cut into wedges

For the tomatillo sauce:

- 4 tomatillos, husked and quartered
- 1/4 cup chopped onion
- 2 cloves garlic, minced
- 1 jalapeño pepper, seeded and diced
- 1/4 cup chopped fresh cilantro
- Juice of 1 lime \s* Salt and pepper to taste

Instructions:

1. Preheat the oven to 375°F.

2. Combine the chili powder, cumin, paprika, salt, and pepper in a small bowl.

3. Brush the fish with olive oil and massage with the spice mixture.

4. Place the fish on a baking sheet and bake for 10-15 minutes or until cooked.

5. While the fish is cooking, create the tomatillo sauce. Mix the tomatillos, onion, garlic, jalapeño pepper, cilantro, lime juice, salt, and pepper in a blender or food processor. Mix until smooth.

6. Warm the tortillas in a pan over medium heat or in the oven for a few minutes.

7. Assemble the tacos by putting a few pieces of cooked fish on each tortilla, topped with shredded cabbage, chopped cilantro, and a teaspoon of tomatillo salsa.

8. Serve the fish tacos with tomatillo sauce with lime wedges on the side for squeezing over the top.

6.10 Grilled pork fajitas

Ingredients:

- 1 pound pork tenderloin, sliced into thin strips
- 1 red bell pepper, sliced into thin strips
- 1 green bell pepper, sliced into thin strips
- 1 onion, sliced into thin strips
- 2 cloves garlic, minced
- 1/4 cup olive oil
- 2 tablespoons lime juice
- 1 tablespoon chili powder
- 1 teaspoon ground cumin
- 1 teaspoon smoked paprika
- 1/2 teaspoon salt
- 1/4 teaspoon black pepper

- 8-10 flour tortillas
- Optional toppings: shredded cheese, sour cream, avocado, cilantro

Instructions:

1. Whisk together the olive oil, lime juice, chili powder, cumin, paprika, salt, and black pepper in a large bowl. Add the sliced pork to the marinade and toss to coat. Cover and refrigerate for at least 30 minutes or up to 8 hours.

2. Heat a grill or grill pan to medium-high heat. Grill the marinated pork strips for 3-4 minutes per side or until cooked through and lightly charred. Remove the pork from the grill and set aside.

3. Heat a drizzle of olive oil over medium-high heat in a large skillet. Add the sliced bell peppers, onion,

garlic, and sauté for 5-7 minutes or until tender and lightly charred.

4. Warm the flour tortillas in a microwave or on the grill for 10-15 seconds to assemble the fajitas.

5. Distribute the grilled pork and sautéed peppers and onions among the tortillas. Garnish with shredded cheese, sour cream, avocado, and cilantro, if preferred. Serve immediately.

6.11 Mango salsa pizza

Ingredients:

- 1 pre-made pizza crust
- 1/2 cup mango salsa (store-bought or homemade)
- 1/2 cup shredded mozzarella cheese

- 1/4 cup crumbled feta cheese
- 1/2 red onion, thinly sliced
- 1/2 red bell pepper, thinly sliced
- 1 jalapeño pepper, seeded and thinly sliced
- 1/4 cup chopped fresh cilantro

Instructions:

1. Preheat the oven to 425°F (218°C).

2. Place the pre-made pizza dough on a baking sheet or pizza stone.

3. Spread the mango salsa evenly over the pizza dough, leaving a 1/2-inch border around the borders.

4. Sprinkle the shredded mozzarella cheese and crumbled feta cheese over the salsa.

5. Add the sliced red onion, bell pepper, and jalapeno pepper to the cheese.

6. Bake the pizza for 12-15 minutes until the dough is golden brown and the cheese is melted and bubbling.

7. Remove the pizza from the oven and sprinkle the chopped cilantro over the top.

8. Slice the pizza into wedges and serve hot.

6.12 Spaghetti with spinach, garbanzos, and raisins

Ingredients:

- 8 oz. pasta (such as fusilli or penne)
- 1 tbsp. Olive oil
- 1 onion, chopped
- 2 cloves garlic, minced

- 1 can (15 oz.) garbanzo beans (chickpeas), drained and rinsed
- 1/2 cup raisins
- 1/2 tsp. red pepper flakes (optional)
- 4 cups fresh spinach leaves, washed and trimmed
- Salt and pepper, to taste
- Grated Parmesan cheese, for serving

Instructions:

1. Cook the pasta according to the package directions until al dente. Drain and put aside.

2. Heat the olive oil over medium heat in a large pan. Add the chopped onion, garlic, and sauté until soft and aromatic for approximately 5 minutes.

3. Add the garbanzo beans, raisins, and red pepper flakes (if using) to the pan and sauté for another 5 minutes, stirring regularly.

4. Add the fresh spinach leaves to the
pan and stir until the spinach is wilted
and soft, approximately 3-4 minutes.

5. Season the mixture with salt and
pepper to taste.

6. Add the cooked pasta to the pan and
toss everything together until the
pasta is covered in the spinach,
garbanzos, and raisin combination.

7. Serve the spaghetti hot, sprinkled
with grated Parmesan cheese.

6.13 Rice noodles with spring veggies

Ingredients:

- eight oz. Dried rice noodles
- 1 tablespoon vegetable oil
- 1 small onion, thinly sliced
- 2 garlic cloves, minced

- 1 cup snap peas, trimmed
- 1 cup asparagus, trimmed and cut into 2-inch pieces
- 1 red bell pepper, thinly sliced
- 1 tablespoon soy sauce
- 1 tablespoon oyster sauce
- 1 tablespoon rice vinegar
- 1 tablespoon honey
- Salt and pepper, to taste
- 2 tablespoons chopped fresh cilantro (optional)
- Lime wedges, for serving (optional)

Instructions:

1. Cook the rice noodles according to the package directions. Drain and put aside.

2. Heat the vegetable oil over medium-high heat in a large skillet or wok.

3. Add the onion and garlic and stir-fry for 1-2 minutes or until the onion is tender and transparent.

4. Add the snap peas, asparagus, and red bell pepper to the pan and stir-fry for 2-3 minutes or until the veggies are tender-crisp.

5. Mix the soy sauce, oyster sauce, rice vinegar, honey, salt, and pepper in a small bowl.

6. Add the cooked rice noodles to the pan and pour the sauce over everything.

7. Toss everything together until the noodles and veggies are covered in the sauce.

8. Garnish with chopped cilantro and serve with lime wedges on the side, if preferred.

6.14 Salad greens with pears, fennel, and walnuts

Ingredients:

- 4 cups mixed salad greens
- 1 big pear, thinly sliced
- 1 small fennel bulb, thinly sliced
- 1/2 cup chopped walnuts
- 1/4 cup olive oil
- 2 tablespoons balsamic vinegar
- 1 teaspoon honey
- Salt and pepper to taste

Instructions:

1. Wash and dry the mixed salad greens and place them in a big bowl.

2. Add the thinly sliced pear and fennel to the salad dish.

3. Mix the olive oil, balsamic vinegar, honey, salt, and pepper in a small bowl until thoroughly incorporated.

4. Drizzle the dressing over the salad and toss lightly to mix.

5. Sprinkle the chopped walnuts on top of the salad.

6. Serve immediately and enjoy!

6.14 Smoky bean and mushroom cornucopia

Smoky bean and mushroom cornucopia is a tasty and satisfying vegetarian meal that's excellent for a weekday supper or a side dish for a holiday feast. Here's a recipe you may follow to create it:

Ingredients:

- 1 big red onion, finely chopped
- 2 cloves garlic, minced
- 8 oz. mushrooms, sliced
- 2 cans of black beans, drained and rinsed
- 1 teaspoon smoky paprika
- 1/2 teaspoon powdered cumin
- Salt and pepper to taste
- 4 big flour tortillas
- 1 cup shredded cheddar cheese
- 1/2 cup salsa
- 1/4 cup sour cream
- Chopped fresh cilantro for garnish

Instructions:

1. Preheat the oven to 375°F.

2. In a large pan, sauté the chopped onion and minced garlic in olive oil until the onion is translucent and the garlic is fragrant.

3. Add the sliced mushrooms to the pan
and sauté until soft and browned.

4. Add the black beans, smoked
paprika, ground cumin, salt, and
pepper to the pan and mixed to
incorporate. Simmer for a few minutes
until the beans are cooked, and the
spices are aromatic.

5. Place one flour tortilla on a baking
sheet and pour a fourth of the bean
and mushroom mixture onto half the
tortilla. Sprinkle a quarter of the
shredded cheddar cheese over the
top of the mixture.

6. Fold the opposite side of the tortilla
over the filling to produce a half-moon
shape. Repeat with the remaining
tortillas and filling.

7. Bake the filled tortillas in the oven for 10-12 minutes until the cheese is melted and the tortillas are crispy.

8. Serve the smokey bean and mushroom cornucopia hot, topped with salsa, sour cream, and chopped fresh cilantro for decoration.

Note: You may add veggies, such as chopped bell peppers, corn kernels, or spinach.

6.15 Spinach and mushrooms frittata

Ingredients:

- 8 big eggs
- 1/2 cup milk
- Salt and pepper to taste
- 1 tablespoon olive oil
- 1 small onion, chopped

- 8 oz. mushrooms, sliced
- 2 cups fresh spinach leaves, chopped
- 1/2 cup shredded cheddar cheese

Instructions:

1. Preheat the oven to 375°F.

2. Mix the eggs, milk, salt, and pepper in a medium bowl until thoroughly blended.

3. Heat the olive oil in a large oven-safe pan over medium heat. Add the chopped onion and sauté until it's transparent and aromatic.

4. Add the sliced mushrooms to the pan and sauté until soft and browned.

5. Add the chopped spinach to the pan and heat until it's wilted and soft.

6.   Pour the egg mixture over the veggies in the pan and swirl gently to spread the vegetables evenly.

7.   Sprinkle the shredded cheddar cheese over the top of the egg mixture.

8.   Place the pan in the preheated oven and bake for 20-25 minutes until the frittata is set and the cheese is melted and golden brown.

9.   Remove the skillet. You may also add other varieties of cheese, such as goat cheese or feta, for a distinct taste.

6.16 Vegetable stir-fry

Ingredients:

- 2 tablespoons vegetable oil
- 1 onion, thinly sliced
- 2 cloves garlic, minced
- 1 inch piece of ginger, peeled and minced
- 2 bell peppers, thinly sliced
- 2 carrots, peeled and thinly sliced
- 1 cup snow peas, trimmed
- 1 cup broccoli florets
- 1 cup sliced mushrooms
- Salt and pepper to taste
- 2 tablespoons soy sauce
- 1 tablespoon sesame oil
- Cooked rice, for serving

Instructions:

1. Heat the vegetable oil in a big pan or wok over high heat.

2. Add the thinly sliced onion to the pan and stir-fry for 1-2 minutes until it softens.

3. Add the minced garlic and ginger to the pan and stir-fry for another minute until aromatic.

4. Add the thinly sliced bell peppers, carrots, snow peas, broccoli florets, and sliced mushrooms to the pan and stir-fry for 3-4 minutes until the veggies are crisp-tender.

5. Season the veggies with salt and pepper to taste.

6. In a small bowl, stir the soy sauce and sesame oil together.

7. Pour the soy sauce mixture over the stir-fry and toss to cover the veggies evenly.

8. Serve the veggie stir-fry hot over prepared rice.

Note: You may add additional veggies, such as baby corn, to the stir-fry. You may add protein, such as tofu, chicken, or shrimp, for a full supper.

CHAPTER SEVEN

7.0 Side Dish Recipes

A renal diet, also known as a kidney-friendly diet, is a meal plan to enable persons with kidney disease or other kidney-related disorders to maintain optimal kidney function. The diet often entails restricting the consumption of specific nutrients, such as sodium, potassium, and phosphorus, while maintaining optimal intake of other nutrients like protein.

Side dishes are integral to every meal, including those on a renal diet. When it comes to picking side dishes for a renal diet, it's crucial to bear in mind the limits and constraints of the diet. For example, many vegetables and fruits are rich in potassium and phosphorus, so it's crucial to pick lower alternatives.

Some solid possibilities for renal-friendly side dishes are steamed or roasted veggies like broccoli, cauliflower, and green beans and salads made with low-potassium vegetables like cucumbers and salads made with low-potassium vegetable lettuce. Alternative possibilities include quinoa, couscous, or other grains that are low in potassium and phosphorus.

Engaging with a healthcare physician or registered dietitian is vital to design a tailored renal diet plan that suits your individual requirements and dietary limitations.

7.1 Mushroom and garlic spaghetti meal

Ingredients:

- 8 ounces of whole wheat spaghetti
- 2 tablespoons of olive oil
- 1 pound of sliced mushrooms
- 4 cloves of minced garlic
- 1/4 cup of low-sodium chicken or vegetable broth
- 1/4 cup of grated parmesan cheese
- Salt and pepper to taste

Instructions:

1. Cook the spaghetti according to package directions until it's al dente. Drain and put aside.

2. Heat the olive oil in a large skillet over medium heat. Add the sliced mushrooms and cook until they release their moisture and brown,

occasionally stirring (about 8-10 minutes) (about 8-10 minutes).

3. Add the minced garlic to the skillet and cook for another minute, stirring constantly.

4. Add the chicken or vegetable broth to the skillet and scrape the bottom of the pan to deglaze any brown bits. Cook for 2-3 minutes until the broth is reduced and slightly thickened.

5. Add the cooked spaghetti to the skillet and toss everything together until the spaghetti is coated in the mushroom and garlic sauce.

6. Sprinkle the grated parmesan cheese over the top of the spaghetti and toss again to mix.

7. Season with salt and pepper to taste.

8. Serve hot, and enjoy!

Note: If you're on a low-potassium diet, you should lessen the number of mushrooms in the dish or swap them with a lower-potassium veggie like zucchini or bell peppers.

7.2 fried rice

Ingredients:

- 3 cups cooked white rice, ideally chilled
- 2 tbsp oil
- 1 small onion, diced
- 1 cup mixed veggies (such as frozen peas and carrots)
- 2 cloves garlic, minced
- 2 eggs, softly beaten
- 2 tbsp soy sauce
- Salt and pepper to taste

- **Optional:** green onions, chopped for garnish

Instructions:

1. Heat a large pan or wok over medium-high heat. Add the oil and stir to coat the pan.

2. Add the diced onions and mixed veggies to the skillet and stir-fry for 2-3 minutes until softened.

3. Add the minced garlic to the skillet and stir-fry for 30 seconds.

4. Push the veggies to the side of the pan and add the beaten eggs to the other side. Scramble the eggs until thoroughly cooked, then combine them with the veggies.

5. Add the cooled cooked rice to the pan and stir-fry for 2-3 minutes, breaking up clumps with a spatula.

6. Add the soy sauce, salt, and pepper to the pan and swirl to mix.

7. Serve hot, garnished with chopped green onions if desired.

7.3 Mushroom asparagus pasta

Ingredients:

- 8 oz of pasta (such as linguine or spaghetti)
- 1 lb of asparagus, trimmed and chopped into 1-inch pieces
- 8 oz of sliced mushrooms
- 2 cloves of garlic, minced
- 1/4 cup of olive oil
- 1/4 cup of grated Parmesan cheese

- Salt and pepper to taste

Instructions:

1. Cook the pasta according to the package directions. Drain and put aside.

2. Heat the olive oil over medium-high heat in a large pan. Add the minced garlic and sauté for approximately 30 seconds until fragrant.

3. Add the sliced mushrooms to the pan and simmer for approximately 5 minutes until they release their juices and become soft.

4. Add the asparagus to the pan and sauté for approximately 5 minutes until they turn tender-crisp.

5. Add the cooked pasta to the pan and stir everything together.

6. Add the grated Parmesan cheese, salt, and pepper to taste. Mix everything until the cheese is melted and everything is properly blended.

7. If preferred, serve the mushroom asparagus pasta hot, topped with more Parmesan cheese.

7.4 Hot chicken penne

Ingredients:

- 8 oz of penne pasta
- 2 boneless chicken breasts, cut into small pieces
- 2 cloves of garlic, minced
- 1/4 cup of olive oil
- 1 can of diced tomatoes (14 oz)
- 1/4 cup of tomato paste
- 1 tsp of red pepper flakes (or more if you like it spicier)

- 1 tsp of dried oregano
- 1/2 tsp of dried basil
- Salt and pepper to taste
- Fresh parsley or basil leaves, chopped (optional)

Instructions:

1. Cook the penne pasta according to the package directions. Drain and put aside.

2. Heat the olive oil over medium-high heat in a large pan. Add the minced garlic and sauté for approximately 30 seconds until fragrant.

3. Add the chicken to the pan and cook for approximately 5-7 minutes until browned on both sides and cooked through.

4. Add the chopped tomatoes, tomato paste, red pepper flakes, dried

oregano, dried basil, salt, and pepper to the pan. Mix everything and bring it to a simmer.

5. Simmer the chicken and tomato sauce for approximately 5 minutes until the sauce thickens slightly.

6. Add the cooked penne pasta to the pan and mix everything until the pasta is covered in the spicy tomato sauce.

7. Serve the spicy chicken penne hot, topped with chopped fresh parsley or basil leaves if preferred.

7.5 Apricot glazed roasted carrots

Ingredients:

- 1 lb of carrots, peeled and cut into sticks

- 2 tbsp of olive oil
- Salt & pepper to taste
- 1/4 cup of apricot preserves
- 2 tbsp of honey
- 1 tbsp of Dijon mustard
- 1 tbsp of apple cider vinegar
- 1/4 tsp of garlic powder
- 1/4 tsp of onion powder
- Fresh parsley, minced (optional)

Instructions:

1. Preheat the oven to 400°F (200°C).

2. Mix the carrot sticks with olive oil, salt, and pepper in a large dish.

3. Spread the seasoned carrot sticks in a single layer on a baking pan.

4. Roast the carrots in the oven for approximately 25-30 minutes until soft and gently browned.

5. In a small bowl, mix the apricot
    preserves, honey, Dijon mustard,
    apple cider vinegar, garlic powder, and
    onion powder until thoroughly
    incorporated.

6. Remove the roasted carrots from the
    oven and sprinkle the apricot glaze.
    Toss the carrots to coat them evenly
    with the glaze.

7. Return the glazed carrots to the oven
    and roast for 5-10 minutes until the
    glaze is sticky and caramelized.

8. If preferred, serve the apricot-glazed
    roasted carrots hot, topped with
    chopped fresh parsley.

7.5 beautiful lemon rice with veggies

Ingredients:

- 1 cup of long-grain rice
- 2 cups of water
- 1/4 cup of olive oil
- 2 cloves of garlic, minced
- 1 small onion, chopped
- 1 zucchini, chopped
- 1 yellow squash, chopped
- 1 red bell pepper, chopped
- 1/4 cup of lemon juice
- 1 tbsp of lemon zest
- Salt and pepper to taste
- Fresh parsley, chopped (optional)

Instructions:

1. Rinse the rice in cold water and drain.

2. Bring 2 cups of water to a boil in a big saucepan. Add the washed rice and a sprinkle of salt to the saucepan. Lower

the heat to low and cover the pot. Cook for approximately 20 minutes until the rice is soft and the water is absorbed.

3. Heat the olive oil over medium-high heat in a large pan. Add the minced garlic and chopped onion to the pan. Sauté for approximately 5 minutes until the onion is transparent and aromatic.

4. Add the diced zucchini, yellow squash, and red bell pepper to the pan. Sauté for 5-7 minutes until the veggies are cooked but still somewhat crunchy.

5. Add the lemon juice and lemon zest to the pan. Mix everything and simmer for another minute.

6. Add the cooked rice to the pan and toss everything together until the rice

is uniformly covered with the lemon and vegetable mixture.

7.   Season with salt and pepper to taste.

8.   Serve the exquisite lemon rice with veggies hot, topped with chopped fresh parsley if preferred.

7.6 Oven-baked green bean fries

Ingredients:

- 1 pound of fresh green beans, trimmed
- 1/2 cup of flour
- 2 eggs, beaten
- 1 cup of seasoned breadcrumbs
- 1/2 tsp of garlic powder
- 1/2 tsp of paprika
- Salt and pepper to taste
- Cooking spray

Instructions:

1. Preheat the oven to 425°F (218°C). Line a baking sheet with parchment paper and gently coat it with cooking spray.

2. Whisk together the flour, garlic powder, paprika, salt, and pepper in a shallow bowl.

3. In another shallow bowl, beat the eggs.

4. Mix the seasoned breadcrumbs and salt in a third shallow dish.

5. Dip a handful of green beans in the flour mixture, brushing off any excess. Then, dip them in the beaten eggs and coat them in the seasoned breadcrumbs.

6. Place the coated green beans in a single layer on the prepared baking sheet.

7. Repeat the dipping and coating procedure with the remaining green beans.

8. Lightly coat the green beans with cooking spray.

9. Bake the green bean fries in the oven for approximately 15-20 minutes, rotating them halfway through until they are golden brown and crispy.

10. Serve the oven-baked green bean fries hot, topped with your favorite dipping sauce.

7.7 chicken and wild rice casserole with butternut squash

Ingredients:

- 1 lb of boneless, skinless chicken breasts, cut into bite-sized pieces
- 1 cup of wild rice
- 2 cups of water
- 1 butternut squash, peeled, seeded, and cut into small cubes
- 1 onion, chopped
- 2 cloves of garlic, minced
- 2 tbsp of butter
- 2 tbsp of all-purpose flour
- 1 1/2 cups of milk
- 1/2 tsp of dried thyme
- Salt and pepper to taste
- 1/2 cup of breadcrumbs
- 1/4 cup of grated Parmesan cheese
- 2 tbsp of olive oil

Instructions:

1. Preheat the oven to 375°F (190°C).
    Grease a big casserole dish.

2. In a big saucepan, mix the wild rice
    and water. Bring to a boil, then
    decrease the heat to low, cover the
    pot, and simmer for approximately
    40-45 minutes until the rice is soft and
    the water is absorbed.

3. Heat the olive oil over medium-high
    heat in a large pan. Add the diced
    onion and minced garlic. Sauté for
    approximately 5 minutes until the
    onion is transparent and aromatic.

4. Add the butternut squash cubes to
    the skillet. Sauté for approximately 10
    minutes until the squash is soft and
    slightly caramelized.

5.   Add the chicken pieces to the skillet. Sauté for 8-10 minutes until the chicken is no longer pink.

6.   In a separate pot, melt the butter over medium heat. Stir in the flour and heat for 1-2 minutes until the mixture is smooth and bubbling.

7.   Gradually whisk in the milk, whisking continuously. Cook the ingredients for around 5-7 minutes till it thickens.

8.   Add the dried thyme, salt, and pepper to the sauce. Mix everything.

9.   Combine the cooked wild rice, chicken, butternut squash combination, and sauce in a large mixing dish. Stir everything together until it is uniformly covered.

10.   Transfer the mixture to the prepared casserole dish.

11.   Mix the breadcrumbs and grated
Parmesan cheese in a separate bowl.
Distribute the mixture evenly over the
top of the casserole.

12.   Bake the chicken and wild rice
casserole in the oven for
approximately 25-30 minutes until the
top is golden brown and crispy.

13.   Serve the chicken and wild rice
dish hot, garnished with fresh herbs if
preferred.

CHAPTER EIGHT

8.0 Dessert Recipes

Renal dessert recipes are created for patients with renal illness who must follow a limited diet to manage their condition. The kidneys play a key function in removing waste materials from the blood. Persons with kidney disease need to be cautious about the foods they consume to avoid placing an additional burden on their kidneys.

A renal diet often entails reducing the consumption of some nutrients, such as sodium, potassium, and phosphorus, while maintaining an appropriate intake of others, such as protein and calories. Desserts may be a tough aspect of this diet since many classic dessert recipes are heavy in salt, potassium, or phosphorus.

Renal dessert recipes typically employ different products or preparation techniques to make tasty sweets that satisfy the nutritional demands of persons with renal disease. Other common components in renal desserts are low-phosphorus milk, egg replacements, and fruits with reduced potassium content, such as apples and berries.

Examples of renal dessert dishes include low-phosphorus rice pudding, strawberry shortcake prepared with low-potassium angel food cake and whipped topping, and frozen banana pops dipped in dark chocolate. These dishes may allow patients with renal illness to enjoy a sweet treat while maintaining their dietary limitations.

8.1 Berries homemade popsicles

Ingredients:

- 1 cup low-potassium mixed berries (such as raspberries, blueberries, and strawberries) 1 cup low-phosphorus vanilla yogurt 1/2 cup low-phosphorus milk one tablespoon honey (optional)

Instructions:

1. Wash the berries and remove any stalks or leaves. Puree the berries in a blender or food processor until smooth.

2. In a separate dish, whisk together the yogurt, milk, and honey (if using) until thoroughly blended.

3. Pour the fruit puree into the yogurt mixture and whisk until well blended.

4. Pour the mixture into popsicle molds or little paper cups.

5. Place the popsicle sticks in the middle of each mold or cup.

6. Freeze the popsicles for at least 4 hours or until frozen.

7. To remove the popsicles from the molds or cups, run them under warm water for a few seconds and gently wiggle the sticks until they come free.

8.2 Pumpkin strudel

Ingredients:

- 1 sheet of phyllo dough
- 1 cup canned pumpkin puree
- 1/2 cup low-phosphorus ricotta cheese

- 1/4 cup chopped walnuts
- 1/4 cup honey
- one teaspoon of cinnamon
- 1/4 teaspoon nutmeg
- 1/4 teaspoon ginger

Instructions:

1. Preheat the oven to 375°F (190°C).

2. Combine the pumpkin puree, ricotta cheese, chopped walnuts, honey, cinnamon, nutmeg, and ginger in a mixing dish. Mix thoroughly.

3. Lay the phyllo dough and brush it with olive oil or melted butter.

4. Spoon the pumpkin mixture over the phyllo dough, leaving a 1-inch border around the borders.

5. Carefully wrap the phyllo dough into a compact cylinder, tucking in the sides as you go.

6. Place the pumpkin strudel on a baking sheet lined with parchment paper.

7. Brush the top of the strudel with a tiny quantity of olive oil or melted butter.

8. Bake the strudel in the oven for 25-30 minutes or until golden brown.

9. Let the strudel cool briefly before slicing it into pieces.

8.3 Delicious cherry cobbler

Ingredients:

- 4 cups pitted sweet cherries

- 1/4 cup honey
- one tablespoon of cornstarch
- 1/2 teaspoon cinnamon
- 1/2 cup all-purpose flour
- 1/4 cup almond flour
- 1/4 cup cornmeal
- 1/4 cup honey
- 1/4 cup unsalted butter, melted
- 1/4 teaspoon salt
- 1/2 teaspoon baking powder
- 1/2 cup low-phosphorus milk

Instructions:

1. Preheat the oven to 375°F (190°C).

2. Combine the sweet cherries, honey, cornstarch, and cinnamon in a mixing basin. Stir thoroughly and transfer the mixture to a baking dish.

3. In a separate mixing bowl, combine the all-purpose flour, almond flour, cornmeal, honey, melted butter, salt,

baking powder, and low-phosphorus milk. Mix thoroughly.

4. Spoon the batter over the cherry mixture, smoothing it out evenly.

5. Bake the cobbler in the oven for 30-35 minutes until the top is golden brown and the cherry filling is bubbling.

6. Let the cobbler cool for a few minutes before serving.

8.4 Little pineapple upside-down cake

Ingredients:

- 1 can of pineapple slices in juice
- 1/4 cup unsalted butter, melted
- 1/4 cup brown sugar
- 1/4 cup low-phosphorus flour

- 1/4 cup almond flour
- 1/2 teaspoon baking powder
- 1/4 teaspoon salt
- 1/4 cup low-phosphorus milk
- one egg
- 1/2 teaspoon vanilla extract

Instructions:

1. Preheat the oven to 350°F (175°C).

2. Drain the can of pineapple slices, retaining the liquid.

3. Add the melted butter and brown sugar to a mixing dish. Mix well and transfer the mixture to a muffin tin, placing one pineapple slice in each cup.

4. Add the all-purpose flour, almond flour, baking powder, and salt in a separate mixing bowl. Mix thoroughly.

5. Whisk together the low-phosphorus milk, egg, vanilla extract, and two tablespoons of the leftover pineapple juice in another mixing bowl.

6. Add the dry ingredients to the wet components and whisk until blended.

7. Pour the batter over the pineapple slices in the muffin tray, filling each cup approximately 3/4 full.

8. Bake the small pineapple upside-down cakes in the oven for 20-25 minutes or until a toothpick inserted into the middle of the cake comes out clean.

9. Let the cakes rest in the muffin tray for a few minutes before using a knife to loosen the edges and gently remove them.

CHAPTER NINE

9.0 Beverages

If you're following a renal diet, it's crucial to be cautious of the drinks you take as well. Here are some beverage alternatives that are kidney-friendly:

1. **Water:** is the greatest option for keeping hydrated and supporting kidney health. Try to drink at least eight glasses of water every day.

2. **Herbal tea:** Herbal teas, including chamomile, peppermint, and ginger, are terrific alternatives for kidney-friendly liquids. Avoid teas with additional sugar or caffeine.

3. **Low-fat milk:** Low-fat milk is a wonderful source of calcium and protein, but finding a low-phosphorus option is crucial.

4. **Fruit juice:** Fruit juice may be rich in sugar, so picking low-sugar versions like cranberry or apple juice is vital. Avoid citrus juices, which may be rich in potassium.

5. **Lemon water:** Adding a slice of lemon to your water may help add taste without adding sugar or potassium.

6. **Homemade smoothies:** Homemade smoothies prepared with low-potassium fruits like berries and mango and low-fat dairy or plant-based milk might be an excellent alternative for a kidney-friendly beverage.

7. **Limit or avoid alcohol:** Consuming alcohol may be hazardous to kidney health, so it's better to restrict or avoid it completely.

It's vital to consult with your healthcare physician or certified dietitian before making any dietary changes, including your beverage choices. They may make customized advice depending on your requirements.

9.1 Water

Water is vital for kidney health, particularly if you follow a renal diet. Consuming adequate water helps to eliminate toxins and waste products from the kidneys, which is vital for avoiding kidney disease.

Try to drink at least 8 cups (64 ounces) of water daily or as your healthcare physician suggests. If you have a renal illness, your healthcare physician may suggest a certain quantity of water to drink, depending on your unique requirements.

It's crucial to pick the right sort of water as well. Seek bottled or filtered water low in

sodium and other minerals since excessive amounts of these elements
may damage the kidneys. Avoid drinking tap water if it is heavy in minerals like calcium, magnesium, and potassium.

In addition to drinking water, you may also improve your water intake by consuming foods with high water content, such as watermelon, cucumbers, and grapes. These meals help you keep hydrated and promote kidney function.

9.2 Herbal tea

Herbal tea is a fantastic beverage choice for a renal diet. Herbal teas are produced from dried flowers, leaves, and roots of plants and are inherently caffeine-free. They are a fantastic method to remain hydrated without ingesting extra sweets or caffeine.

Some popular herbal teas for kidney health include:

1. **Chamomile tea:** Chamomile tea is a relaxing and tranquil beverage that may help decrease inflammation and promote relaxation.

2. **Ginger tea:** Ginger tea is recognized for its anti-inflammatory effects and may aid in easing digestion.

3. **Peppermint tea:** Peppermint tea is a delicious and soothing drink that may help ease an upset stomach.

4. **Hibiscus tea:** Hibiscus tea is a tangy and delicious beverage that may help decrease blood pressure and reduce inflammation.

5. **Dandelion root tea:** Dandelion root tea is a bitter drink that may help improve digestion and decrease inflammation.

While picking herbal teas, it's crucial to check the labels and avoid beverages with added sugars or artificial flavors. It's also crucial to consult your healthcare physician or qualified nutritionist before introducing herbal teas to your diet since certain herbs may interact with specific drugs or have other health concerns.

9.3 Low-fat milk

Low-fat milk is an excellent beverage choice for a renal diet since it delivers key minerals like calcium and protein without adding too much phosphorus, which may damage the kidneys. Calcium is vital for keeping healthy bones and teeth, while protein is needed for developing and repairing structures in the body.

When buying low-fat milk, it's crucial to find a low-phosphorus alternative. These may include skim or 1% milk, which have less phosphorus than higher fat milk variants.

You may also pick plant-based milk substitutes like almond or soy milk, but reading the label and choosing a low-phosphorus is vital.

Checking your portion amounts while ingesting low-fat milk is vital since it still includes some phosphorus. One serving of low-fat milk is normally 1 cup (8 ounces), so be conscious of how much milk you take throughout the day.

If you have kidney illness, it's vital to speak to your healthcare practitioner or registered dietitian about your unique dietary requirements and how much low-fat milk you should take daily.

9.4 Fruit juice

Fruit juice may be a healthy beverage choice for a renal diet, but it's crucial to pick the correct kinds of juice and be aware of the amount.

When picking fruit juice, it's vital to choose low-sugar choices since excessive sugar may damage kidney health. Excellent alternatives for low-sugar fruit juice are cranberry or apple juice. It's also vital to avoid citrus liquids like orange or grapefruit juice since they are rich in potassium, which may be hazardous to persons with renal illness.

It's vital to note that fruit juice is still heavy in sugar and calories, so monitoring your portion sizes is crucial. One serving of fruit juice is generally 4 ounces or half a cup. It's also a good idea to dilute your juice with water to minimize the sugar level and keep you hydrated.

In general, it's better to take whole fruits instead of fruit juice since they are lower in sugar and fiber. If you want to eat fruit juice, it's vital to do so in moderation and as part of a balanced renal diet.

9.5 Lemon water

Lemon water is a popular beverage choice frequently claimed for its health advantages, particularly its ability to assist kidney function. Yet, it's crucial to recognize the possible hazards and advantages of drinking lemon water if you have kidney illness or are following a renal diet.

Lemons are a strong source of vitamin C, an antioxidant that may help protect against kidney damage. They are also natural diuretics, which may assist in improving urine flow and washing out toxins from the kidneys.

Nevertheless, lemons are also strong in citric acid, which might raise the risk of getting kidney stones. If you have a history of kidney stones or are at risk of getting them, you must check with your healthcare professional before taking lemon water.
Also, it's crucial to understand that lemon water is acidic and could harm tooth enamel over time. To lessen the danger of tooth damage, it's a good idea to sip lemon water via a straw and rinse your mouth with water after drinking.

If you have kidney illness or are following a renal diet, it's vital to consult with your healthcare professional or qualified dietitian before adding lemon water to your diet. They can help you assess whether it's safe and acceptable for your unique requirements.

9.6 Homemade smoothies

Homemade smoothies may be a nutritious and pleasant beverage alternative for a renal diet. You can manage the ingredients by creating your smoothies and guarantee they are kidney-friendly.

While creating a smoothie, picking low-potassium and low-phosphorus fruits and vegetables is crucial. Some nice selections are berries, apples, pears, cucumbers, and leafy greens like spinach or kale. You may add protein to your smoothie using low-fat yogurt or nut butter.
Checking your portion sizes while ingesting smoothies is vital since they may be heavy in calories and sugar. Go for a serving size of 1 cup and avoid adding additional sugar or sweeteners.

This is a simple recipe for a kidney-friendly

Smoothie:

- 1/2 cup fresh or frozen berries
- 1/2 medium apple, peeled and diced
- 1/2 cup chopped cucumber
- 1 cup fresh spinach
- 1/2 cup low-fat yogurt
- 1/2 cup water or unsweetened almond milk

Blend all ingredients in a blender until smooth, and enjoy!

Suppose you have kidney disease or are following a renal diet. In that case, it's important to talk to your healthcare provider or registered dietitian about your dietary needs and how much fruit and vegetables you should consume daily.

9.7 Limit or avoid alcohol

Individuals with kidney disease are generally recommended to limit or avoid alcohol consumption. This is because alcohol can negatively affect the kidneys and worsen existing kidney damage.

The liver processes alcohol, but excessive alcohol consumption can cause liver damage and increase the risk of liver disease. This can also impact kidney function, as the kidneys rely on the liver to process waste products and toxins.

Moreover, alcohol may promote dehydration, which can be hazardous to renal function. The kidneys are crucial for controlling fluid balance in the body, and excessive alcohol intake may upset this equilibrium and contribute to dehydration.
If you want to drink alcohol, it's vital to do so in moderation and as part of a balanced renal diet. This often involves reducing alcohol intake to one drink per day for ladies and no more than two drinks per day for males. It's also vital to pick low-potassium and low-phosphorus alcoholic drinks, such as light beer or wine.

Suppose you have kidney illness or are following a renal diet. In that case, it's vital to speak to your healthcare practitioner or registered dietitian about your unique dietary requirements and how much alcohol you should eat daily. They can help you assess whether it's safe and acceptable for your unique requirements.

CHAPTER TEN

10.0 Meal Planning

A renal diet, often known as a kidney diet, is a specific meal plan for patients with kidney disease or decreased kidney function. The purpose of a renal diet is to lessen the stress on the kidneys and treat symptoms such as fluid retention, high blood pressure, and electrolyte abnormalities. These are some basic recommendations for meal planning on a renal diet:

1. **Limit sodium:** Sodium may promote fluid retention and high blood pressure, damaging the kidneys. Avoid processed and packaged meals rich in salt; pick fresh, natural foods instead. Reduce your salt consumption to fewer than 2,300 mg per day.

2.   **Monitor protein intake:** Protein is vital for maintaining muscle building and facilitating recovery, but too much protein may damage the kidneys. Check with a nutritionist to establish the optimum quantity of protein for your unique requirements.

3.   **Choose low-potassium foods:** Potassium is a mineral that may collect in the blood when the kidneys are not working correctly, leading to muscular weakness, irregular heartbeat, and other issues. Select low-potassium foods such as apples, berries, grapes, cabbage, green beans, and cauliflower.

4.   **Avoid high-phosphorus foods:** Phosphorus is a mineral that may build up in the blood when the kidneys are not operating correctly, weakening bones and creating other difficulties. Avoid high-phosphorus foods such as

dairy products, processed meats, and carbonated drinks.

5. **Drink lots of water:** Keeping hydrated is vital for kidney function and may help drain toxins out of the body. Drink lots of water throughout the day, and avoid sugary or caffeinated drinks.

It's crucial to talk with a qualified dietitian who can help you build a tailored food plan that suits your particular requirements and interests. They can also help you monitor your nutritional consumption and make modifications as required.

10.1 Establishing a Weekly Meal Plan

This is an example of a one-week meal plan for a renal diet:

Monday

- **Breakfast:** Scrambled eggs with low-potassium veggies (such as spinach and peppers), whole-grain bread, and a small slice of low-sodium bacon.

- **Lunch:** Chicken and vegetable stir-fry with brown rice.

- **Dinner:** Grilled salmon with roasted asparagus and a tiny baked sweet potato.

Tuesday

- **Breakfast:** Oatmeal with sliced apples and cinnamon.

- **Lunch:** Turkey and avocado sandwich on whole-grain bread, served with a side of baby carrots.

- Dinner: Roasted chicken breast with steaming green beans and quinoa.

Wednesday

- **Breakfast:** Greek yogurt with low-potassium fruit (such as berries) and granola.

- **Lunch:** Low-sodium turkey chili with a side of whole-grain crackers.

- **Dinner:** Spaghetti squash with low-sodium marinara sauce and turkey meatballs.

Thursday

- **Breakfast:** Spinach and feta omelet with whole-grain bread.

- **Lunch:** Tuna salad with low-sodium crackers and cucumber slices.

- **Dinner:** Grilled pork tenderloin with roasted Brussels sprouts and wild rice.

Friday

- **Breakfast:** Banana and peanut butter smoothie prepared using low-potassium components.

- **Lunch:** Grilled cheese sandwich with low-sodium tomato soup.

- **Dinner:** Baked salmon with steamed broccoli and a small dish of whole-grain couscous.

Saturday

- **Breakfast**: Spinach and mushroom frittata with whole-grain bread.

- **Lunch:** Chicken and vegetable soup with a side of whole-grain crackers.

- **Dinner:** Stir-fry meat with low-potassium veggies (such as bell peppers and onions) and brown rice.

Sunday

- **Breakfast:** Whole-grain pancakes with low-potassium fruit (such as blueberries) and a small amount of low-sodium sausage.

- **Lunch:** Grilled chicken salad with low-potassium vegetables (such as lettuce, carrots, and cucumbers) (such as lettuce, carrots, and cucumbers).

- **Dinner:** Baked tilapia with low-sodium roasted potatoes and steamed green beans.

Remember to work with a trained dietitian to design a tailored meal plan that suits your particular requirements and tastes. They can also help you monitor your nutritional consumption and make modifications as required.

10.2 Grocery Shopping Tips

Suppose you follow a renal diet; picking the correct items while grocery shopping is crucial to preserving kidney health. Here are some guidelines to help you make the correct choices:

1. **Plan:** Create a shopping list before you go to the supermarket. This will help you avoid purchasing needless things and ensure you have all you need for your renal diet.

2. **Choose fresh fruits and vegetables:** Fresh fruits and vegetables are a fantastic source of nutrients and are low in sodium and potassium. Opt for fruits like apples, cherries, and grapes and veggies like broccoli, carrots, and kale.

3. **Look for low-sodium options:** Select low-sodium versions of meals such as canned veggies, soups, and broths. Check labels carefully to be sure you are not receiving too much salt.

4. **Choose lean protein sources:** Choose lean protein sources, including chicken, turkey, fish, and tofu. They are lower in phosphorus than red meat.

5. **Limit processed meals:** Processed foods like chips, canned products, and packaged snacks are generally rich in salt and phosphorus. Minimize your consumption of these items and opt for fresh, healthy meals instead.

6. **Drink lots of water:** Keeping hydrated is vital for kidney health. Drink lots of water throughout the day and avoid sugary beverages like soda.

7. **Consult with a certified dietitian:** If you need clarification about which foods to eat, speak with a registered dietitian who can give individualized suggestions based on your unique requirements.

By following these recommendations, you may make healthy choices while food shopping for a renal diet.

10.3 Planning Meals in Advance

Preparing meals in advance is a terrific way to save time and guarantee that you have nutritious, kidney-friendly meals accessible throughout the week. Here are some recommendations for preparing meals in advance for a renal diet:

1. **Plan your meals:** Before you start cooking, plan your meals for the week. This will assist you in ensuring that

you have all the ingredients you need and can prevent wasting food.

2. **Choose kidney-friendly dishes:** Look for recipes low in salt, potassium, and phosphorus. There are several websites and publications available that specialize in kidney-friendly cooking.

3. **Cook in batches:** Prepare large amounts of food at once, then divide the portions into containers for later use. This may save you time and make it simpler to keep to your renal diet.

4. **Store food properly:** Keep your cooked meals in the fridge or freezer in airtight containers. Label them with the date, so you know when they were made.

5. **Reheat properly:** While reheating your meals, follow food safety requirements. Reheat food to at least 165°F (74°C) and stir periodically to ensure equal cooking.

6. **Use convenience foods:** If you need more preparation time, seek healthy convenience meals like pre-washed and pre-cut fruits and vegetables, canned beans, and low-sodium soups.

7. **Experiment with flavors:** Just because you're following a renal diet doesn't mean your meals have to be boring. Experiment with herbs, spices, and other ingredients to flavor your food.

By preparing meals in advance, you may save time and make it simpler to keep to a kidney-friendly diet.

10.4 CONCLUSION

A renal diet cookbook may be a valuable resource for anybody following a renal diet. It can inspire new recipes, offer guidance on which foods to avoid and which to incorporate, and make meal planning and preparation easier.

When choosing a renal diet cookbook, look for one tailored to your specific needs, such as one for people with kidney disease or one focusing on low-sodium, low-potassium, and low-phosphorus recipes.

It's important to remember that while a renal diet can be challenging, eating delicious, kidney-friendly meals with the right ingredients and preparation techniques is possible. A renal diet cookbook can help you start this journey and be a valuable tool for maintaining kidney health.

www.ingramcontent.com/pod-product-compliance
Lightning Source LLC
Chambersburg PA
CBHW070823250726
48662CB00003B/1069